CW01512956

SELLING 1
AS PODIATRY

Promoting your service to patients

David R Tollafield

A Reflective Podiatric Practice Series

Busypencilcase Reflective
Communications
Cover design by Andy Meaden

ISBN: 9798641635118

Established 2015

THE SINGLE BIGGEST PROBLEM WITH
COMMUNICATION IS THE ILLUSION THAT IT HAS
TAKEN PLACE

GEORGE BERNARD SHAW

The following material was developed from a series
of Reflective Articles published for podiatrists
during 2019-20

Books by the same author
(*available from Amazon*)

Podiatry & Foot Health

Clinical Skills in Treating the Foot, Churchill-Livingstone with Linda Merriman

Assessment of the Lower Limb, Churchill-Livingstone with Linda Merriman

Morton's Neuroma. Podiatrist Turned Patient: My Own Journey.
A New Foot Pain Series

Bunion. Hallux Valgus. Behind the Scenes.
My Patient Journey Series

Professional Skills

Presenting Your Image
Conferences to Village Halls

Thinking as We Build
PowerPoint is More Than a Slide Programme

Children

The Story of Cristal Rouge
(as Rob C Blyth)

Foreword

In the United Kingdom the Foot Health Market is valued in many millions and yet Podiatry practice accounts for only a tiny percentage of that market. The share by professional practice is small even when you include NHS and private practice.

One has only to spend a couple of hours watching commercial television to view advertising for footwear, fungal skin and nail treatment, bunions, corn cures, orthotics, insoles, electrical treatments, verrucae and many others to realise that for large corporations selling foot health direct to the public is big business. Add in social media, radio and print and it becomes possible to wonder how a small business private practitioner can make a living let alone a good profitable income.

Standing out in this crowded world sets the tone to convince the patient population that self-diagnosis is not the best way to deal with foot health issues and then paying out money for good treatment. Paying for treatment when the UK population expects most healthcare to be free at the point of delivery adds another barrier.

Starting out in private practice is a daunting prospect. Single handed or multidisciplinary, high street or house conversion, bank loan or equipment rental? These and many other questions have to be faced by the new entrant to podiatric private practice. What are you providing, a service certainly, but are you also selling skills and probably prescribed items? How do you value what you have?

I would hope that attitudes have moved on from the 1980s when I was refused a bank loan to buy a thriving practice for the reason that the business had too little stock to be viable. The bank manager said that no value could be placed on my skills and the patient numbers attending the practice.

Now new practitioners have to deal with social media, websites, and advertising. They have to understand the power of branding and reaching their potential patient populations. I recommend this book to all new podiatry practitioners and to those looking to improve their practice marketing. The author takes you through the various stages of learning how to brand your practice and fight your way to success.

If I had seen this book at the start of my career I would have avoided mistakes and been well placed to succeed in the 21st century practice world.

Ralph B Graham
Past Chairman, College of Podiatry

Preface

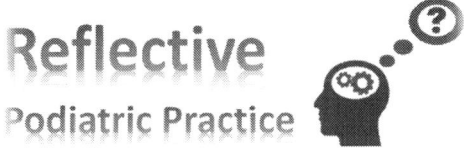

A bit of reflection

During my working life I listened to some of my erudite colleagues say, *'when I retire I will start to write'*. I have come to learn that it is not easy to write if this is something not carried out during one's career. This is certainly true when writing is not a natural part of one's occupation. Originally I tried to write for my grandchildren. My first book was called *The Story of Crystal Rouge* when the world of self-publishing first looked attractive. I used what is called Vanity Press. In this scenario there is limited control of your product once launched and costs related to all the production stages soon mount up. Then it comes to the point where you are charged per page. The story idea was credible but the book was a flop in terms of sales. Vanity Press created too many constraints. I had failed to appreciate 'marketing and design' and felt I was throwing good money away. This meant I could not communicate with the outside world because I could not promote my message. It was a pivotal moment for me. Continue, or give up! I chose to diversify, change direction and take control. Giving up was not an option.

Most sales techniques are about finding the right market place and with podiatry we need to resonate with foot conditions and attract related subjects. This book is not about writing but the subject of promotion and communication. What gets you out of bed each day and what motivates you must drive your interest and enthusiasm. My ability at self-branding as a podiatrist proved more successful than the branding of my pen name, Rob C Blyth, which being an unknown was another part of the problem.

Without giving away too much, as practitioners of the art and science of foot health we hold in our purview a subject that goes back to the 18th century. The foot health professional often fails to create sufficient impact upon the health market. Surgeon chiropodist, Lewis Durlacher made his own mark and created a brand known even in Royal circles. In today's multi-faceted world of high speed communication and competition we need to use any tool at our disposal.

My own brand as a podiatric surgeon was easy as I was hooked into an automatic referral system through the GP network, but that was aided by decades of working within the NHS which sold my product (me) and the delivery of foot health consultations for patients referred by their GPs.

Those first years in private practice set in a small Midlands town were painfully slow and caring for my new family meant watching the pennies. Diversifying into biomechanics, as it was branded then, kept the wolf from the door as locum work only just paid the mortgage!

You might be forgiven in thinking that this book is just about making a living, but it is as much about promoting the subject of podiatry. The work of Professor Catherine Bowen and a project called *OptiFoot* brings into focus not just how we are seen as podiatrists but how patients are failing to connect to the most appropriate services within the NHS. Readers are therefore reminded that branding, promotions, education and communications are not isolated to private independent practice alone but involve one of the biggest brands in the market place, *the NHS*.

Communication between colleagues, and patients provide an important platform for your services. It is hoped that for those wanting to kick start a career in podiatry, or in practice already, are made aware of the obstacles affecting our profession and the delivery of the message as to who we are and what we do. There is no better place to start than with an article written following a series of talks based on communication given to a number of podiatry branches in England. I have expanded the subject based on concepts embraced by the work of Silverman and colleagues. Examples and some anecdotal experience are shared from my own practice and some discussion is given to modern forms of supporting verbal communication.

Tony Gavin (OSGO) provides helpful material covering business and his thoughts on branding in chapter 1. Elsewhere I look to Sonia Gregory (Freshsparks) who offered some illumination into the concept of branding and can be reached through her website and then there is a useful book by Catherine Kaputa (2012) '*You are a Brand'* that guided some of my own reflective thoughts throughout.

It is hoped that the material within **Selling Foot Health as Podiatry** is of value to all, even non-podiatrists, and that it contains some useful anecdotes that bear fruit.

Promoting our professional business is fascinating and it has been fun dipping into the subject of podiatry that has remained the corner stone of my life.

**David Tollafield,
May 2020**

www.consultingfootpain.co.uk
davidt@busypencilcase.com

Contents

Acknowledgments

I am indebted as usual to others who have willingly given their time to be my guardians of the written word. This book was only going to be a 1/3rd of the size it is; a thin morsel built from articles written for colleagues. It turned out to be anything but as natural curiosity accumulated and I delved deeper into the subject.

To engage beta readers, copy editors and proof readers is a vital part of an author's supportive team. The author generates the ideas and writes them down but without the wisdom of independent people the writer's creation can suffer from a sense of misalignment, ambiguity, being partisan and idealism.

Sidney Gibson has been invaluable having an eye for creative advertising. Although a non clinician he was able to view the narrative from a layman's point of view. Tony Gavin, while my junior accumulated more knowledge around formal business than I and so leaning on his experience was welcomed. His vision of podiatry is infective, not least because he had many useful thoughts that I have injected into this book.

I am also indebted to the wonderful work that Professor Cathy Bowen and her team have achieved around their OptiFoot project. Providing additional material from an NHS perspective was important.

NHS podiatrists should now view their business differently.

Ralph Graham represents an enduring professional clinician and foot surgeon with 50 years' experience. Having worked within two titled organisations[1] and acted as a clinical manager both in the NHS and Private Practice, who better to overview my proselytizing method.

Ralph was the first to reassure me that my own independent practice, which commenced in 1981, would take five years to become established, in that he was correct.

Andy Meaden put together a great cover for this book with that difficult final decision assisted by a number of podiatry colleagues who continue to also act as great beta readers.

Thank you for your ideas, kind assistance and words of wisdom which I hope have sewn seeds to mitigate my own errors.

---

[1] Podiatry Association and The Society of Chiropodists & Podiatrists (College of Podiatry)

1. What's in a name?

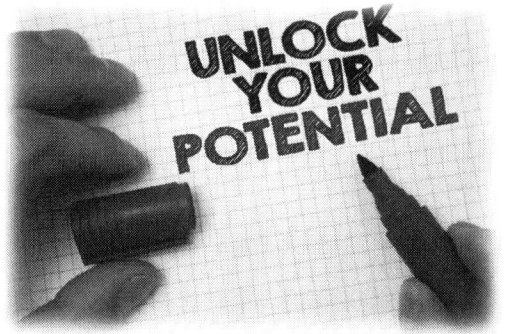

Shutterstock/Artur Szczybylo

From Squire to Knighthood, Mister (Mr) or Miz (Ms) to Professor, we all aspire to have some type of nominal. My father still writes 'Esq.' at the end of my name on the envelope with the correct avoidance of Mr at the front end. Esquire is used when addressing a person who has a post-nominal professional designation but not both. Esquire is a courtesy title and has its origins steeped in medieval Europe although Parker defined it in 1894 as a title of rank. The French word *escuyer* comes from shield and is tied up with rank below a Knight.

It is doubtful many would use Esq. today which can in fact include all genders. We are wedded to titles and even those who leave military service retain commissioned service titles usually at the level of Major or above in the UK.

The different titles within podiatry have been expanded with extended scope podiatrist, specialist podiatrist, consultant podiatrist, all attributed to different interests and service delivery. The use of titles often considers how we feel others perceive us as much as how we perceive ourselves, a little like medals and letters of merit bestowed by Royal decree. I have not knowingly observed a podiatrist with letters used for financial gain, but in general people use titles and post nominal letters to show they are learned. Most titles are used within polite conversation as part of respect. Inevitably we will use titles within our business and initiate who we are and what we stand for. Professionals trained in a specific field of study find it much easier to convey the nature of their role within a short sentence. And so whether we work in the NHS or independent sector we will use title, rank, designated employed title to demonstrate what we do which in turn links to our responsibility. Outside larger institutions all these ways of expressing ourselves pale into insignificance when we step into the independent sector. Armed with our most essential qualification that allows us to register for practice, it is 'US' and how we function that matter.

We are professionals but also business people who provide a service. It is clear that we must understand what a business is but also optimise who we are. There are numerous books on business and help can be acquired through the internet and its vast resources, but when it comes to the specific nature of our business we can drill down a little further. The NHS is a business but we probably don't see it as that as individuals, but lean on the NHS brand to speak for itself. Alone and away from big brand names it is just us.

THE NAME OF THE BUSINESS

As with many professions, the terminology associated with practice can be confusing. For most people reading this book, you may have had a brief association with the word chiropody. Where the two titles i.e *chiropody/podiatry* are used together the ambiguity of terminology can confuse the objective behind defining what service is actually being provided.

Some people suggest that there is no difference between these titles but it could be argued that in fact the difference is not just philosophical but functional. As providers we might wear several hats, but an opaque image is counterproductive.

So how did all this confusion come about?

The field of foot health was formerly known as chiropody up until 1988 and then it became not just confusing, but more confusing. Lewis Durlacher[2] (1792 – 1864) had used *surgeon chiropodist* during his working career in the 19th century. A small number of Chiropodists formed a special interest group in surgery and adopted the title podiatry in 1975, at the time formalised by examination (MPodA). The term podiatry was imported from the USA where US podiatrists wanted to prevent confusion with chiropractic and chiropractor and subsequently changed their title in 1958. This provided a significant opportunity to rebrand their profession which they did successfully. Podiatry in the USA is protected in title and in functional delivery which means you cannot treat feet unless qualified as a doctor of podiatric medicine (DPM).

In circa 1988 the UK profession converted their primary qualification from *diploma* (DPodM) to *degree* (BSc Podiatry) and changed the course title to podiatric medicine or podiatry, replacing the subject of chiropody. In 2018 the Society of Chiropodists & Podiatrists dropped their title,

---

[2] Durlacher held the appointment as Surgeon-Chiropodist to the Medical Department of the Royal Household of King George IV, King William IV and Queen Victoria. On one occasion he demonstrated his operation for ingrowing toe-nail at the Hospital of Surgery in Panton Square, London.

originally incorporated in 1945 as the Society of Chiropodists, and then again in 1996-7, and became the College of Podiatry. The Institute of Chiropodists & Podiatrists did so likewise but retained the title chiropodist within its overall title in 1995. The original group called podiatrists adopted the title Podiatric Surgeon because GPs had become used to the term podiatry, implying 'surgery' and chiropody as 'non-surgery'. The podiatric surgeon required entry to practice by rigorous examination and a university based course for the didactic elements which incorporated a pre fellowship MSc Podiatric Surgery (circa 2003-4).

In 2003 the Council for Professions Supplementary to Medicine (CPSM), including the Chiropodist Board, was changed to the Health Professions Council (HPC) then again later to the Health & Care Professions Council (HCPC). This Government statutory body protects standards of practice in patient care delivery with defined sets of practical and theoretic skills supporting each qualification and group on its register. The HCPC has expanded from its original remit and now incorporates fifteen professional groups at this present time. The HCPC restricts the use of title rather than ability to practise foot care. Foot care assistants and Foot Health Practitioners (FHPs) provide allied services but do not come under the HCPC and are disallowed from using the terms podiatrist and chiropodist.

And so your title is likely to be associated with podiatrist or podiatry, or podiatric medicine, the latter being more attuned with newer attitudes. So schools of podiatry also became schools of podiatric medicine. With degrees the schools morphed into departments within Health Faculties. What you call your self is one thing, but what you present as the face of your business is another.

Professor Cathy Bowen has been working on a large project called *OptiFoot* as well as closely with the Arthritis and Musculoskeletal Alliance. She says

> Some patients are still confused with our terminology and that's from a profession that evolved over the last 30 years that has evolved from being chiropodists to what is now termed podiatry. And that still causes endless confusion with people because they think these two are different, when in fact they are not because this was a name change, and it is the fact that the podiatrist scope of practice has advanced so much over the last 30 years that the two are quite distinct. But some people still retain the name because they are frightened of losing the people that still go to see them and that understand what chiropody is. (2019)

In 1980 the title British College of Ophthalmic Opticians (Optometrists) was adopted. In 1987 the title was changed to British College of Optometrists and in 1995 the title College of Optometrists was adopted. If you look at the College of Ophthalmic Opticians little is discussed about a change of name, but in the high street the older optician title has all but disappeared. 'Op-' as a prefix occurs in both names, and yet elsewhere there is a suggestion that another group have used the title optician as in *dispensing opticians*.

An Irish group called Eyezone has published this explanation;

> The official definition of Optometry is a long one! Basically, it is the study of primary eye and vision care. The field of Optometry has become extremely vast in the past 30 years, and naturally, branches began to form in the field. The most widespread of these is the Dispensing Optician. Most people simply use the word "Optician" for everyone in the field, which is not strictly correct. Historically, we were all simply called Opticians. You may still see the words "Ophthalmic Optician" on some older premises. The historical term for "Optometrist" was "Ophthalmic Optician". An Optometrist is trained to provide eye and vision care, performs eye examinations to detect vision problems, and prescribes corrective lenses to correct those problems. Most Optometrists also make and fit spectacles. Optometrists are trained to fit contact lenses, and to provide complete aftercare for them. In Ireland, an Optometrist is not a medical doctor, and cannot prescribe medications. An Optometrist can provide eye exercises and dry eye treatments. When an optometrist detects eye disease, the patient may be referred instead to an Ophthalmologist, a physician who specialises in evaluating and

treating diseases of the eye. A Dispensing Optician is person trained to make and fit spectacles. They do not perform eye exams or fit contact lenses. Dispensing Opticians are fully trained and qualified to provide advice on the best type of spectacle frame and lenses for a patient, once the spectacle prescription has been determined. Technologies over the last couple of decades has made lens and frame choice extremely vast. This is where the Dispensing Optician comes in. Some Dispensing Opticians choose to study further, and some also become contact lens opticians or low vision specialists. So, there are many kinds of Optician: Optometrist (Ophthalmic Optician), Dispensing Optician, Contact lens Optician, Low Vision Specialist… and many other areas of Optometry left to be explored!

http://www.eyezone.ie/content/whats-difference-between-optometrist-and-optician. Accessed April 2020. Eyezone are a large company promoting the brand of optometry and optometrists.

THE CONUNDRUM OF LANGUAGE

Add to the confusion of name used by eye specialists to that of ophthalmic surgeon or ophthalmologist and we see more confusion. And so Podiatry is not alone but the words C- and P- do add to problems. In the case of pharmacies and chemists, where both have a different first letter *P&C*, they haven't suffered to any great extent. Both are consistent brands that exist within high street stores offering other healthcare products. Language is complex and to change brands requires great thought. For those of many years in age, chemist was the name while pharmacy probably came about with the inclusion of the UK into Europe. In reality the explanation is more complex. Chemists make up chemicals and are scientists while pharmacists are health professionals who dispense medicines. In 1953 the Pharmacy Act came into being under pharmaceutical chemists. So this is how name changes become confusing. Coming back to chiropody versus podiatry one can see that the language of what we call ourselves does not make it any easier when the HCPC still use chiropodist alongside podiatrist.

WHAT IS A BUSINESS?

'The definition of business is a systemised exchange of value. It introduces service or a product into the market. The provider of that service and the recipient of the product exchange money, goods or actions, so that both leave with more than they came with.

This is what business comes down to when stripped of all jargon. If everything that happens in a business is reliant upon your action or decision alone, then I would suggest that you have not created a business. This is because you have to become the business directing it so that it can work and develop on its own. The term director comes from giving direction. It's sitting at the top of the mast on the ship and pointing that's the way we are heading. If you are down on the wheel or moving the sails about all of the time, it is very difficult to see and direct where that ship is going.

We think that a big part of our identity is the ability to do it all and that it doesn't extend to running businesses. There is an expectation that we can run a business as podiatrists. However, while this is true to a point, and while there's a huge amount of advice and support available, nothing replaces the value of experience in running a business. Just like clinical practice requires self reflection on a regular basis, it also requires having a mentor who can challenge you and constant pursuit of improvement.

We massively undervalue what we do as podiatrists. Most practices will survive because they'll be able to meet rent and put food on the table. There are so many foot problems out there that most practices, if they tick enough of the boxes of being in the right location, and being open for the right number of hours, and have an appropriate price point, will survive.

That doesn't mean that it is a good business. Surviving in business for 5, 10, 20 years is not necessarily the sole measure of success. A successful business goes through constant growth. It's not just financial growth but growth in what it's delivering to the 'world'. It may niche down and implement more technical services or something similar that matters to the business owner. Business therefore must constantly grow and improve. The other question to ask is, if you are the business yourself, if there are no system policies and procedures or updated documents in place then is it a business?' (Gavin 2020).

These enthusiastic words from a podiatrist and businessman conducted by interview cover structure, key features of business acumen gathered from nearly a decade of experience before entering the profession of podiatry, and after successfully running other businesses. For the readers who now have knowledge and a license to practice, we still have to promote ourselves to drive our business. Tony Gavin concludes,

'It is pretty difficult to open a podiatry practice and not survive because the income is relatively strong compared to many other people trying to run businesses. However, it is easy to lose income by making bad decisions from performing badly.'

In some way the success of many of our decisions comes back to our image. People's perception of our ability which contributes to the brand which is really US.

In chapter 2 we move into the arena of the clinic, face to face contact with the client (patient) and experience the subject of communication.

2: Communication with Patients

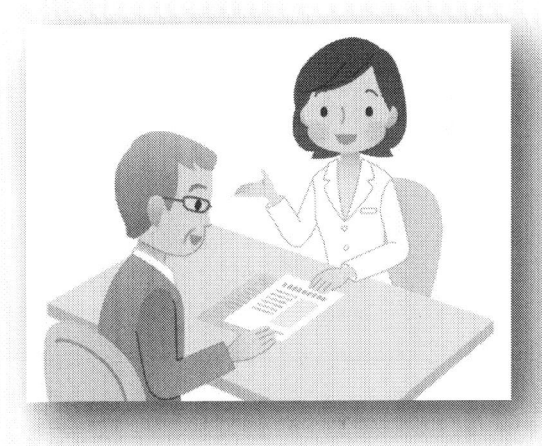

Shutterstock / Kotikiti

It has been acknowledged that the amount of time given to listening to patients before interruption is, on average, under 18 seconds (Beckman & Frankel 1984). The evidence for this is strongly highlighted in publications, but as a phenomenon amongst medical doctors this is hardly new. When attending a medical communications day at the King's Fund Institute some years ago this important element of communication was the first to be discussed. In contrast, the series 'GP Behind Closed Doors' on Channel Five was often an eye opener. Take away all the excellent care and knowledge in a busy UK practice, some GPs were still falling into this age old trap of short circuiting the patient's ability to finish their opening complaint. So it still goes on!

We are all patients at some time in our lives. While still working I had access to a network of medical care and my GP knew me for well over 25-years as both podiatrist and patient. His time keeping was poor as he was frequently late. Should I judge him by the criteria as a bad GP? NO. First of all, his patients all had different problems and needed different time allocation. And, he always listened first. After I moved to a new area I saw three different 'consultation faces' at my new GP practice. The one that resonates with me most was a forty something male GP who candidly told me that if I wanted to discuss a second item (which incidentally related to the first), then I needed a second appointment. I responded with raised hackles,

> *'You GPs do have a problem with time!'*
> *'You can always book a 20-minute*
> *appointment next time if you want*
> *longer,'* he replied.

How much time should we allow for consultation?

It is GPs not the Government that determines the time of consultation. As a clinician I recognise patient problems come in all shapes and sizes. Their problems often can be solved quickly, for some however more time is needed.

So how long should we allow a patient to talk?
Back to the King's Fund Institute communications course in London; if you let a patient talk uninterrupted they will more often stop talking within 150 seconds. For the GP and a 10-minute rule that is taking up 25% of his self imposed allocated slot.

> GP appointments should be extended to 15 minutes because an ageing and increasingly overweight population means that many patients need extra time at the doctors' surgery, according to the British Medical Association (BMA).
> The standard slot currently stands at 10 minutes but the BMA GPs committee (GPC) believes that increasing the length of appointments by 50% would allow for improved decision-making and service, as well as reducing the administrative burden for doctors outside clinic hours. (Guardian 2016)

'The Ibuprofen Model'

Some patients leaving surgeries in the *Channel Five programme* are being put into a convenient holding bay. The 'ibuprofen model' of care is similarly axiomatic for pain problems affecting the foot. It is available by self purchase, avoids a prescription and is cheap. It provides both analgesic and anti-inflammatory properties so why criticise this approach?

Without carefully taking a good history covering drug habits and sensitivities one can cause the patient side effects, worse still affect the heart or gastrointestinal systems. A limited period of use for such a drug is important. Three days' worth should allow determination that a condition is being helped. Three weeks without review hardly constitutes good care. The patient does not need to return in 4 days but should be aware that if the drug does not help then it should be discontinued. If the drug is beneficial then an adjunctive strategy is worthwhile such as rest, ice and maybe some form of splinting. If benefit and response fail, then new strategies should be adopted including diagnostic screening to cover differential diagnosis. To most podiatrists this would all seem obvious, to the GP who is the first line clinician it seems more than ever that their actions relate to managing a busy caseload.

Calgary-Cambridge Model

Making comparisons between medical doctors as the face of healthcare may seem unreasonable when compared to podiatry. In general, podiatry has traditionally allowed 20 minutes for what was known as routine care delivery. With the advent of the musculo-skeletal examination in the late 1970's and known as a biomechanical examination, the time rose as additional methods were added. The consultation for the podiatric surgeon in my own practice would usually cover a 25-minute slot, although the allocated slot for efficiency for NHS patients was 15-20 minutes. It was not unusual to use 40 minutes for new consultations. Jonathan Silverman together with co-authors Suzanne Kurtz and Juliet Draper criticise the medical model of clinical assessment, Silverman et al (2013).

Their aim was to improve doctor-patient care. While recognising the good elements of medical care, there were glaring flaws in the healthcare model that had been considered clinician centred.

The usual introductory greeting might be *'How can I help you?'* Better still a rephrased greeting sets the scene and clarifies the goals immediately.

'What do you want to achieve from your consultation?' can be slipped in. You now have a contract that can be documented.

After years in practice reaching a rapid diagnosis does become easier but care always beckons us to not reach a hasty conclusion. The anecdote of a young podiatrist keen on 'biomechanics' in 1978 demonstrated an easy weakness in less experienced podiatrists. In this case the podiatrist failed to take an adequate history or basic skin examination. Having flipped the patient into a prone position, he suddenly admitted with some embarrassment that the problem was a verruca and that the newly acquired skill of biomechanics was not required. Taking a clinical history still counts, but will have little value if we fail to listen. Eyes on the computer will remove direct contact from the patient and so we miss the non verbal cues.

The Root of All Complaints

Patients are often frightened, an emotion easily missed. Patient focus means that we have to provide measured information that can be understood, digested, reasoned with to make a decision. The days of the patient leaving it to the G.P. doctor has disappeared into the sunset. Even the well healed phrase, *'What would you do if it was your foot?'* is a less ideal method to respond when a patient glibly asks of the clinician their view through personal experience. Seeking a glimmer of direction for themselves is understandable and difficult to resist.

The perimeter of 'financial inducement' is often claimed as a complaint, and one to be avoided. This is difficult for some working in the NHS where a decent budget may not be available but where advice can direct a patient to make a self-pay purchase directly to another source. However, a boundary will have been crossed if clinicians direct NHS patients to their own private enterprising practices. Despite this appearing to help the patient, and maybe well meaning, disciplinary action rarely sides with this ethos.

Modern independent practices possibly, emanating from dental practice, require all costs to be provided in a clear unambiguous way. This is a good development for those paying for a service.

Misunderstanding is the root of most clinical care complaints and even litigation. Communication is now a science because we can apply quality research tools to acquire better comprehension. Social media needs to be factored into communication as exposure to additional information is made possible before the patient arrives at your door. The study of patients' wants and needs has been suggested through a UK study where 55% of patients wanted specific treatment, 60% had their own ideas and 40% focused on concerns about their symptoms (McKinley & Middleton 1999).

Clearly each patient has a different agenda and it is the skill of the clinician who can identify this need. The ideas that patients foster about their treatment and care will come from better patient awareness of their body. Once the domain of female patients, male patients, especially those of the generation 30-40 group may well have researched the field more than their older male counterparts. The questions asked are more direct than those of older generations and might well be more forceful. This is a positive not a negative change and allows the clinician to focus on patient fears and need. What is best for the patient has to be seen from both sides of the problem. Using clinical knowledge and careful communication, the patient presented with equal options will change their mind. On many occasions GP letters would state,

> *'…the patient does not want surgery.'*

After a consultation some patients would change their mind. This was not because of any passion to undertake surgery, but because the solutions available could only lead to a realistic cure which was more cost effective than conservative care.

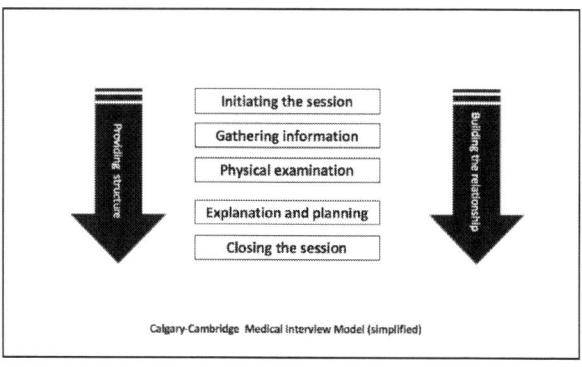

Figure 1
Basic Framework Calgary-Cambridge Model adapted from Silverman et al (2013). Burt et al (2013) describe a rating scale based on this model

In his paper on hammer toe surgery, Hood (1991), then a podiatry student, looked at conservative versus surgical management of digital deformities and exemplified the point about economical benefits to the patient. Sometimes surgery is better justified than endless repetitive care. Our duty is to advise patients on best practice but with a clear eye on respecting their preference.

Silverman developed the joint Calgary-Cambridge approach to patient communication as far back as 2007. Having used this as a basis for talks on patient communication I decided to distil their version highlighting the desirable elements of a patient interview without going into detail. The basic framework of the medical interview per Silverman however is still important (Figure 1) as it included the standard medical approach with a patient sensitive involvement as a scheme.

The physical examination follows the standard processes seen in healthcare while the other 4 elements (in Figure 1) make a subtle departure.

Choice – Knowledge – Action – Understanding – Reassurance (C– K.A.U.R)

A mnemonic C-KAUR helps to navigate five principles that we can derive from the Calgary-Cambridge Model and adapt for podiatry or any clinical consultation process. This is then embedded within the business model for promoting our consultation aims

Choice

Patients must have choice to decide what level of help they require and this should be made clear early on. The remainder of their preference will be developed through the remaining elements. While coercion is unlikely, it can be implied and the risk of complaint or even litigation can find barristers attempting to use lack of choice as a breech of appropriate consent.

Knowledge

The provision of information about the condition should take into account the patient's wishes and aims of why they attended your clinic. The sharing of knowledge and listening is vital to the plan. Foot management needs to meet both their physical (organic) and their socio-economic requirements.

Action

Forms the treatment plan and will concentrate on the elements associated with 'patient can do for themselves', supportive treatment and specific treatment only delivered by podiatry intervention. The outcome of action must be shared. I have used the Ibuprofen model earlier to highlight some of the dangers of non-shared action with the patient, i.e what is the next stage to offer some inclusive knowledge?

Understanding

Choice is underpinned by understanding the condition together with any implications behind any decision. Meeting the requirements of patient driven decisions can only be achieved by sufficient discussion of any benefit versus risk versus effectiveness. Not every patient wants the type of management that a clinician feels appropriate and so (s)he must be careful not to appear coercive.

Reassurance

The closure of the session between patient and clinician is as important as the initiation. Trust between the parties is vital to ensure the best compliance. Patients may be just as happy with *doing nothing* as have *something done*. When they leave clinic they should feel as though they have had good value from their consultation. The objectives stated at the start of the clinical interview should ideally have been met, and that the patient feels that they have been listened to.

Focusing on What Matters

Optimising on the principles of good communication with our patients will drive more referrals and broaden recommendations to the business. Despite all the efforts in promoting your service; self-referrals and those recommended by others will be based on the very qualities that you bring to your face-to-face consultations with patients.

Clean lines, uncluttered rooms, a clear recognition of instrument sterilisation and friendly staff cannot be underestimated. The location and design of the practice plays an ever increasing draw for patient clients. Of all the qualities podiatrists can offer, providing the time to listen, using empathy and integrity together with appropriate onward referral when needed will trump all other promotional cards in the pack.

Patients warm to honesty and appreciate saving money without the hard sale. For any other country in the world this may be different but the British public put their trust in those that exude trust.

3: How to communicate

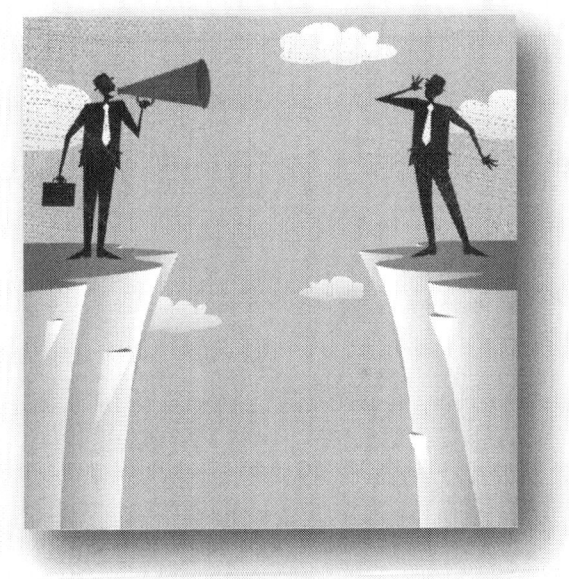

Shutterstock/ Jorgen Mclemon

RECORDING THE REAL NEEDS OF THE PATIENT

The podiatrist is taught to undertake a clinical interview, examination, plan and execute a treatment using the format of *subjective, objective, assessment and plan*, reduced to the the abbreviated forms SOAP or recently SOAPIER (Cowley 2018). This mnemonic has been the focus on how to take a clinical history and examination since the seventies and was embroidered into a system called the National Record Card. The Association of Chief Chiropody Officers (ACCO) promoted the A4 format in favour of the postcard system. The relevance to us was the importance of accounting for more detail and appearing to adopt a clearer medical model. The postcard system became a Lloyd-George format but was marred by the use of unintelligible hieroglyphics and the overuse of the ditto mark. In today's terms any legal case would soon determine this practice substandard.

Recording information is as important to show a plan of activity as it is to communicate between colleagues and teams. By 1990 the podiatric surgery team at Northampton School of Podiatry introduced the US American method of the history and physical (H&P) that expanded on the SOAP method. This closely allied to the UK system called clinical clerking as used by medical students (Seymour C, 1984). Today H&P is still in vogue and broken down into the body systems (Kilmartin et al, 1991).

Both the SOAP and H&P amount to the same thing, and yet the depth of the interview and examination may vary and *red flags* may be based on different scopes of practice. Missing the queues associated with the patient's true concern arises because they feel historically a need to be led and it is only the stronger patient that resists this so called tug of war. Consultation periods within the private healthcare market tend to be longer and have a direct correlation with different forms of funding.

Surgery v. non surgery

Doctor knows best attitude is a dangerous precept and as Beckman & Frankel (1984) found, words and questions from the clinician can inadvertently direct the patient away from the real reason for being at the consultation (Silverman 2013). In many cases the podiatrist has a referral and the patient is focused on one aspect of footcare. However, take the case (Tollafield 2018) where a patient had bunion pain without realising some of the focal pain came from a digital neuroma. The neuroma was more difficult for the patient to understand than the bunion, and yet dealing with both was required. This particular case history ended up with litigation and *communication* was part of the critical element of claim against the podiatrist. The patient denied understanding any part of the consultation! The judge ruled in favour of the podiatrist and believed the misunderstanding unlikely. This clinical situation is rare and not a true reflection following most consultations. The podiatric surgeon, a clinician who acts in the sense of tertiary care as opposed to the podiatrist more often acts within secondary line care, generally takes his lead from a clinical referral. Patients often appear from other sources with recommendations for surgery. There have been occasions when inadvertent surgery is carried out because of the assumption that this is what the patient wants. Adopting a new line of questioning can avoid this phenomenon. The initiation of the interview must set the parameters as suggested earlier.

> *'Your GP has referred you for surgery. Is this what you want?'* [Clinician]
> *'I know he mentioned surgery but no I don't really want surgery!'* [Patient]

Orthotic management

Podiatrists wanting to use orthotic management are placed in similar positions of responsibility and the financial package may often appear as costly as some surgeries. The duty of care extends to quality communication about 'action'. The decision must be shared and based on good understanding and knowledge (education) of the condition.

A case of a patient in 1981 who was persuaded to have an orthotic prescription fell off a roof and was invalided and so could not afford the device. The podiatrist had to meet the laboratory costs as the patient refused to pay.

The patient argued that he had not understood what the device was and thought it to be a shoe! This exemplifies two problems. Orthoses produced by laboratories were new in 1981. There was no insurance to cover this type of eventuality. The podiatrist while well meaning might not have selected a prescription orthotic which cost £43.00 to his practice. A simpler orthosis might have been wiser. This was a case of jumping a stage. *That clinician was me!*

Most of the consultation is based on two people facing each other using words, facial expressions and body movement to project meaning. Understanding cannot be assumed from facial expressions alone. Memory recall varies between patients and key words are vital to trigger emphasis of each point. Here is a typical scenario:

> Clinician: *There are risks associated with this treatment that might leave you worse off.*
> Patient*: I can't be worse off than I am now!*

Impairment

Hearing and understanding are also two different elements that make up positive or negative communication. A patient with poor hearing will fill in the blanks, often processing information inaccurately.

Receiving bad news alters the state of memory. Someone who is told they have a malignant lesion on the foot may block all information. While words are important, podiatrists should use other methods to reinforce communication.

ADJUNCTIVE METHODS OF COMMUNICATION

Aid-memoires are valuable for communication. Five methods are discussed although not all may be relevant.

Models
Patients who handle the bones of the foot are fascinated by the relationship of this complex anatomical structure. Holding and examining a foot can help reinforce verbal explanation. While bones highlighting joints and positioning have value, sometimes plastic models with cut out sections to show anatomy are worthwhile.

Diagrams
It is worth having books and leaflets with diagrams or separate pictures to show patients. Good quality photographs or line drawings are helpful to allow you to discuss different aspects of pathology. Patients can be directed to a personally preferred website for further information provided that they are in agreement, but this should be documented.

E-methods and drawings

We are not all artists and one big problem is scale and relationship within drawings. Stick diagrams are effective but clarity helps. Its is possible to acquire free and for purchase, pre drawn material that makes life easier which patients can take away. My preference was the newer concept digital tablets that you can draw on as well as write on, noting the patient's name and date. These can be printed off using a wifi connected printer or sent to the patient as well as having the advantage of keeping the information stored in your records.

Leaflets

Leaflets can be purchased and of course save time in a busy practice, but personalised leaflets will always carry greater gravitas. Highlighting information is valuable and can be used as a significant reference helping patients to make decisions. The take away value is important as it provides a patient with the all important aid-memoire. Patient leaflets can be time consuming to produce. The downside to any leaflet or written information is that it must be kept in date and consistent with other practices.

Film

There can be nothing more valuable than a well made film, one with good direction and illustrations. Film (video) can be selected by YouTube and most subjects can be found. There are caveats. The narration must be clear and without heavy accent. While British English is best for UK patients there are some excellent American English films on foot problems. Nick Campitelli's short film covering neuroma lasts 0.39 minute. This illustrates a quality example of video.

Film should always be checked first before being recommended. The time should be around ½ to 4 minutes in length and no longer for essential information based on one theme. The advice and information should be clear, non fuzzy and free from excess gore.

Surgical film should ideally carry some type of warning. My own information sheets for patients from my website have embedded film. The downside is that some links can be lost as the linked material may have been removed, often inadvertently after being updated. Any means you use to support communication should ideally be checked regularly to ensure it still works. Conversion to Portable digital files (PDF) can also remove hyperlinks

Websites
Websites[3] are valuable tools and are usually employed to direct business. One of the better websites that extols the value of podiatric work is that of Ivan Bristow providing multiple options for promotion and communications. The website is

---

[3] Websites cited in this chapter were all accessed between 2019-2020

probably not intended as much for patients as for clinicians owing to its higher academic content.

Another website example associated with promotion of podiatry is by Dean Walsh from the Midlands. This site forms the other end of the spectrum. The advertising covers simple information about podiatric conditions and would suit patients.

The Exeter clinic website contains a useful home page with conditions and information where the factsheets are summarised and therefore brief. In contrast, ConsultingFootPain[4] is different as there is no practice, and it focuses on patient information and Journey experience, but embedded with clinical experience.

While there are many examples of websites for podiatrists they all have an expiry date and constant maintenance is necessary. While I have selected three excellent examples randomly, all accessible by internet search, many podiatrists will have spent time and money in developing a robust programme of information that not only promotes podiatry but offers quality information. While all patients can be invited to use websites (also see chapter 11), it is essential that patients have the option for hard copy which may require larger words for those with impaired site and macula degeneration. It is

---

[4] The author's website ConsultingFootPain is an information based resource centre helpfully linked to support the public and podiatrists.

important to appreciate that not everyone has abilities with information technology (IT).

The End of the Interview

Closing the patient interview is as important as the opening process. Doctors appear good at clarifying the plan (75%) but poor at checking understanding (34%). Orientating patients to the next step and providing information falls to 56% and 53% respectively White et al (1994). The values given show the frequency taken from listening to audio tapes at closure. Understanding the element of risks has always been valuable. Using known data in any form of promotion can be powerful. Eight reports, between 2010 and 2017, show a mean of 97.8% confirmation of understanding risk about surgical treatment (97.5-98.2)[5]. Podiatry is more likely than not to perform better than medical practices because it invests more time in patient contact. But, in the end it comes down to the quality of the delivery that counts.

Conclusion

Patient choice in making decisions and the need to ensure that we listen to their needs becomes an essential part of the consultation based on the Calgary-Cambridge method of modelling. Care

---

[5] College of Podiatry PASCOM-10 system of clinical outcome measurement data collection. www.pascom-10.com

must adopt a shared process considering the need to check understanding of any knowledge imparted that impacts on the plan. C-KAUR provides a simpler model although does not take the place of the detail found within the Calgary-Cambridge system. Podiatry can offer better communication to patients than many GPs who still operate a formal model in the arena of information delivery.

Communication is a skill, an art and a science and honing best methods are essential for health care delivery. The quality of that communication can be enhanced by observing best practice based on evidence. As always in our field nothing stands still. Before we can form the basis of a business we must recognise that communication skills make up an internal process.

The external process contributes to the remaining emphasis within this book and ensuing chapters but must not negate from the importance of engaging with patients directly when they arrive at our clinic. How we interact with patients affects our success when delivering our brand. It is easier to promote ourselves once we have a patient, but there is still the skill in attracting patients to make that appointment.

In the next chapter I will cover aligning information with promotional value as well as discussing what conditions are presented by professional bodies

4: Information conversion

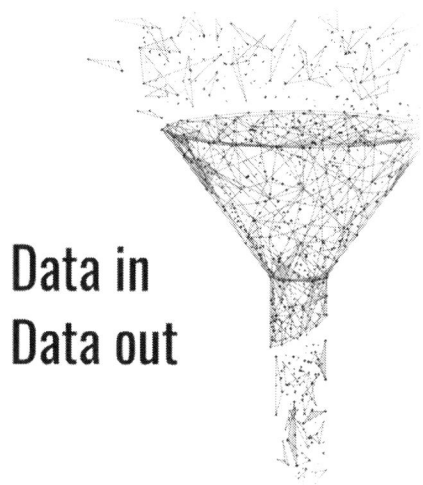

Data in
Data out

SCIENCE AND POLICY

I wrote to Michael Harrison-Blount and congratulated him on his recent paper in the Journal of Foot and Ankle Research (JFAR, 2019) and posed the question that had been nagging at me ever since JFAR had grown in strength. Science uses formal narrative. How far do we use formal science before we confuse our patients with complicated?

language associated with the structure of academia versus lighter conversation? Michael's paper provided me with some reflection on the complexity of evidence and how it reads and is consequently understood.

If we write papers with an academic rigour, interpretation should translate the message without ambiguity in order for successful implementation. It should be added that it is not necessarily the academic author's role to bring this change. If one person lights a firework, someone else might see to its safe delivery. But who's responsibility is this?

Look at the way in which politicians used the scientific material to drive policy during the pandemic coronavirus attack in the first quarter of 2020. The chief scientific officers were trying to provide evidence to drive policy decisions. The politicians knew if they stuck close to scientific recommendations any shortfall might be reviewed more favourably.

Given that the media has qualified health journalists with scientific backgrounds, it was clear that during the crisis, shortened to Covid-19, that social media and mixed interpretation arose before all the data could be analysed and then translated for reliable consumption. The outbreak will become an enduring example of communication and information conversion.

Primordial Cascading

As a profession we have worked hard to create an academic degree based profession. And yet for every clinician there is a reader. For every reader who is a clinician there is a patient. For every patient there is a need to transmit information at a comprehensive level. How we transmit information can alter the interpretation of the meaning, if not the gravitas behind that message. There are two premises that drive primordial cascading. The first is communication, the second is dealing with a changing landscape or progressive development of therapeutic scope of practice. The two are inevitably linked.

Harrison-Blount published the idea of changing landscapes affecting podiatry and could only find answers when delving into the publications from other professions. This we can call evidence. So often, in order to make headway, the researcher has to run a parallel enquiry as nothing is as it seems. And so, if the landscape is changing, it might have had little leverage from podiatric literature where no such citations exist.

Farndon, a podiatrist keen on the study of epidemiology in podiatry probably comes as close as any to giving us numbers and attitudes, Farndon (2006). The literature forms the basis of evidence and evidence drives decisions. *Or does it?*

How do we convey any shift in clinical attitudes and practice to our patients, and perhaps beyond them to our public? We publish of course. But what do we publish and where should we publish for impact, and how complicated does the material need to be to be taken seriously?

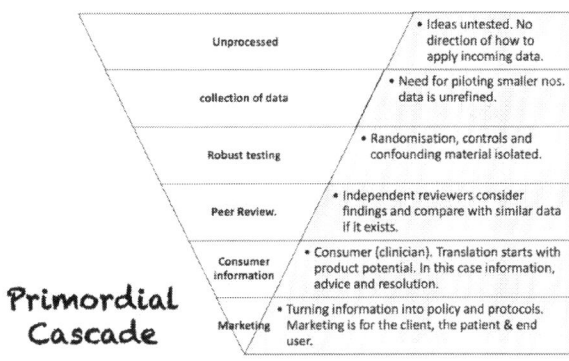

Figure 2

Primordial cascade demonstrates that there is a hierarchy in the way that information is translated then converted into marketing strategy.

It is often axiomatic that the more complex a subject the less appeal it will have upon a broad readership within the idea of it being understood. It is not until the consumer level is achieved that this top down approach to informative material provides the ideal narrative to assist patients.

Harrison-Blount's academic paper is not hard to read, it has depth and breadth, but it needs interpretation. This is where there is an unspoken problem. Where only a small part of a profession read beyond general information. Academic structured articles remain more common within set courses and training cultures where such material is mandated. There has to be a reason to read such material. This carries no intended criticism, or indeed a desire to dilute progress since the first 4-year degree courses were developed in London c.1985, beyond the Open University structure used by early podiatrists for academic development. Those who perform research and write measure in small numbers, judging by our publication output. To communicate we must reach the consumer to drive podiatry business.

Is Podiatry a business?

'If we are to drill down to the core of communication, it comes down to a business proposition.'(Gavin 2020).

We have a commodity and require our public to buy into our product. Our product is foot health provision; diagnosis and management. Management broadly implies how we organise and administer the delivery of a service. The services we offer are broadly advice, self help, conservative intervention and restoration of function.

Other professions will compete. Forty years ago had this been discussed within our baseline education the attitude would be; we are not salespeople and to be so would demean us. We are professional and at that registered! Today this approach would appear old fashioned.

Being professional does not mean that we cannot advertise as long as we are truthful and the material is accurate. Being registered is not a qualification, it is a mandatory requirement that reflects that we meet minimum standards to practice behind the word podiatry. We know that registration is not functional so others can treat the foot but should not use the term podiatry (and chiropody) as a representative title. Misleading the public is an often banded phrase used by detractors. The Registry that retains on record podiatrists under the Health and Care Professions Council does not promote us. Ironically it will pillory us if we transgress over self aggrandised promotion. Afterall it is the guardian of part of the health market.

Categorically podiatry is a business and the greater proportion of podiatrists are in the self-employed sector. So who markets us? Former podiatrist Jill Woods says on her website,

> My job is to cut through the clutter & the waffle, giving you what you need, to get to where you want to be, in as short a time as possible.

She is an inspirational healthcare marketing coach and listening to her at the NEC healthcare conference in 2019 demonstrated her astute awareness that damage can arise from labelling blame. So when as clinicians we blame poor publicity on any named group, we are not taking responsibility.

Practices promote themselves avidly, driving patients toward a programme of care. This is positive but most websites promote the business not healthcare per se. Afterall to promote too much free material could detract from that all important income. There is a growing philosophy though that the more you profile yourself, the more you gain acceptance. Give aways drive promotion and business your way.

How do we package a product?

As an author, communicator and self styled foothealth journalist, I can see with better clarity how we might develop our promotional platform. It involves a dynamic shift taking on a new functional appearance. That appearance requires a better association with medical models.

The pre-eminence of a profession comes from recognition invoked by statute initially, and the legal framework that allows you to do something with permission by society. One needs to provide evidence that we do 'good', but who says what good is? Good comes from standards and expectations of performance laid down by others.

The barriers to change have been summarised as resistance. But where does this resistance come from? As Harrison-Blount puts it, '*it is the organisation, the profession and service level users*'.

The impact from our changing work force practise has toppled many previous held thoughts about autonomy. In the NHS there is a drive toward multidisciplinary teams or MDTs. Changes within this large employing body however has seen shrinking numbers of podiatrists attracted to full-time NHS employment. Furthermore, the attraction toward a career in podiatry is not as healthy as it should be. It has been intimated that the fault lies with the policy in regard to educational grants and financial support. There is no doubt that that being able to afford to study for 3 years requires some investment, but is this truly the whole reason for demise?

MARKETING AS A CONCEPT

Podiatry offers a good career and should be an inspiration, and yet it does live in a quagmire of identity confusion. The career structure is not without its attractions and delivering foot health care is very rewarding. But how do we package care and footcare? Well it comes back to marketing your

brand which essentially is you. That marketing has to be clear and targeted. Harrison-Blount says the demand is high and that a ¼ of the population will reach age 65 by 2033 which suggests a figure around 18 million. That premise could suggest that we are required to provide for those over 65. This has been the focus of organisational policy for ½ century, and certainly applied to the NHS care delivery.

Private practice attracts those who are not funnelled into such historical categories, but then how far can the NHS budget stretch? I predicted in 1983 that podiatric surgery would not be able to offer surgery for bunions. We are still delivering this service because of need and inequalities elsewhere. So, it could be that we have filled a need. Being useful drives business as it has value, until it doesn't or it is too expensive. Diabetic care, and those with at risk conditions take priority beyond the traditional groups. In the NHS this has extended the product line for NHS podiatrists.

Where does resistance come from?

Resistance comes from the organisation and profession. Who is the organisation and profession if it is not us? Polarised attitudes by a small group of people can make a difference and this is seen as a problem. A profession that has no competition thrives but domination also stifles beneficial development. Such was the case of the podiatry profession during the 50s and 60s when a determined group wanted to see an expansion of service delivery. The case for dentistry having no identity crisis is predicated by their dominance in a field that even medicine does not routinely touch. Contrast this with podiatry and competition has been growing.

Statistics

What once might have appeared a stable approach to podiatry is no longer so stable. Two key professional bodies exist in the UK offering membership. Both produce websites and it is upon national websites that image is created because of accessibility. Granted a percentage of the population neither have the skills or preference for the internet platform but this is dwindling year on year. Compare two years of Office for National Statistics (ONS). Government statistics suggest that in 2016, while 99.2% of adults aged 16-24 used information technology by 2019 adults aged between 16-44 showed 99% use. By 2019 adults between 16-74 showed that 95% were recent users, the third highest in the European Union.

There has been a steady growth of disabled users with 10 million recorded in 2019. Adults aged over 75 showed the lowest group of users at 38.7% in 2016 which grew to 47% three years later. London and the South East suggest the highest group internet users in the population. Data still might not account for the devastating effect of aged macular degeneration so figures are subjective in some cases.

Business is about consumerism, and demand creates a shift in decisions as to what to sell. Why do people come to podiatrists? Is it for palliation or a cure? The latter would seem to be the more significant objective, although we recognise the pampering effect amongst the population is gender dominant. However, professional websites punch out the message *condition*. But what conditions do they promote?

Taking patient information from each of the 3 UK sites[6] dedicated to Foothealth (Table.1) it is possible to see the main foot health areas promoted.

Top Foot Health Conditions

The top conditions (Table 1) include athletes foot, corns and callus, fungal infections, heel pain, sports medicine, arthritis, children's foothealth advice. Diabetes and bunion are the only subjects common to all three groups. Table 2 shows patient accessible information.

---

[6] College of Podiatry, The Institute of Chiropodists & Podiatrists and the British Orthopaedic Foot and Ankle Society. Links to each of these organisations are provided in the reference section at the end of the book.

College of Podiatry	Institute of Ch. & Podiatry	British Orth.Foot & Ankle Soc. BoFAS
Ageing feet	Corns & calluses	Arthritis foot and ankle
Athletes foot	Verrucae	Sports injuries
Blisters	Excessive perspiration	Fractures in the foot and ankle
Bunions	Bunion Hallux valgus	Foot problems in diabetes
Chilblains	Athletes foot	Birth deformities
Corns & calluses	Tips caring for your feet in sport	Heel pain
Gout	Footcare for diabetics	High arched feet
Heel pain	Fungal infections of the nail	Flat feet
Ingrowing toe nails	Orthotics	Bunions
Osteo-arthritis	Suggestions for healthy feet	Problems with small toes
Rheumatoid arthritis	Care for babies and small children	
Sweat feet		
Verrucae		

Table 1

Relative comparison between three dedicated UK foot websites.
[Accessed 04/2020]

College of Podiatry	Institute of Ch. & Podiatry	British Orth.Foot & Ankle Soc. BoFAS
Keep on walking	Public resource links	Achilles tendon
Footwear	Corns & Callouses	Hallux valgus
Sports med. (incl. shoes)	Verrucae	Hallux rigidus
The patient's perspective	Bunions (Hallux Valgus)	Flat feet
Advice for parents	Athletes Foot	Heel pain
Diabetes	Caring for your feet during sport	IGTN
	Footcare for diabetes	Metatarsalgia
	Orthotics a modern way to prevent foot & leg pain	Ankle arthritis
	Some suggestions for healthy feet	Lesser toes
	Footcare for babies & small children	Cavus feet
		Ankle instability

Table 2

Relative comparison between three organisations and
available literature cited from individual websites

Do opinions from a different profession affect podiatry?

The BoFAS site which is an orthopaedic interest group has members from the orthopaedic community who publicise their views about 'chiropodists' often avoiding the word podiatry. Snap shots of how one profession attempts to change the market impression of another profession can be successful if it is not challenged effectively.

Statement #1

> Chiropodists will generally offer treatment for problems of the skin and nails of the feet, and some are trained in the production of special insoles to improve foot function and comfort.

Statement #2

> Basic chiropody training includes very simple surgery, such as the toenails. Some chiropodists, or podiatrists, study surgical techniques further and may offer surgical treatment for various conditions. The place of this type of service has not yet been established.

The first statement informs the public about the role noting that '*will generally*' is active not passive, in relationship to a podiatrist's main interest. When statement #1 is read in terms of '*some are trained in the production of special insoles...*' the (BoFAS) author fails to acknowledge that insoles and prosthetic theory and practical elements are the mainstay of podiatry undergraduate courses. This may be from chairside to in laboratory workshop management as well as taking of casts. The second statement fails to clarify nail surgery or place it into any correct perspective. There is no such matter as simple surgery but misleading titles as 'simple' elevate the opinion inadvertently or deliberately to demean the work of another.

The high nail regrowth rate following nail surgery was the very reason that podiatry adopted the principle role of managing *all things nail*. Dr Clare Laxton, an independent researcher, published a cross professional paper. Nail surgery really looked good in the hands of podiatrists and poor in the hands of surgeons but equivocal when it came to digital lesser toe surgery, Laxton, C (1995).

Evidence can often discredit bias or self gratifying opinions and it is a reminder to anyone publishing or promoting health that it is unhelpful trying to achieve an advantage over another person just because you can. In another statement BoFAS posed the question, *can chiropody help with deformed toes?*

Statement #3
> A chiropodist can give advice about shoes and insoles, and can treat the hard or raw skin that develops over some deformed toes. Chiropodists in Britain and most parts of Europe do not operate to straighten toes

In this third statement BoFAS suggested that '*Chiropodists… do not operate to straighten toes*' This is only accurate in relationship to the fact that podiatrist is the preferred term and chiropodists do not straighten toes but **some** podiatrists **can**.

In the second paragraph '*the place of this type of service has not yet been established,*' is inaccurate in some ways and accurate in others. This means that it is divisively ambiguous. Progress in surgery has taken 45 years to create a well defined structure which will almost certainly be regulated at the highest level when the HCPC with the support of the GMC establishes a new register[7]. It serves to remind us *that terminology acts as the gravy to nourish words but is often manufactured to alter the taste by the cook but not by the restaurant* (author).

In any other respects adverse publicity, as seen in tabloid press between 2008-2014 is often inaccurate and misdirects the reader to believe something that may not be quite true but has just enough leverage to suggest concern. Despite being briefed by the former College of Podiatry, The Society of Chiropodists & Podiatrists, the publicity department and two other Deans, on 2nd July 2012 Louis Rogers for The Daily Mail misled the public as to the length of podiatric surgical training.

Lawrence Ambrose wrote in Podiatry Now (2020), the College of Podiatry's main newsfeed to its members.

> The extent of what podiatrists do and can do 'isn't recognised in the wider healthcare system as much as it should be'.

As Head of Policy and Public Affairs he would be aware how others view the profession and yet persuading organisations such as BoFAS to change

---

[7] Registration of British Podiatric Surgery is at an advanced level of annotation at the time of writing this book.

their representation of podiatry seems to remain a challenge surrounded by diplomacy? Ambrose goes on to say that 'Podiatrists are taking a lead in clinical care...'. In the same article the undisclosed author, assumed the editor, Emma Godfrey, suggests that;

> One of the primary aims (*of enhancing understanding*) is to make it clear to the public that podiatrists are experts in all aspects of the foot and lower limb.

Susan Knight, a Queen's Nurse specialises in tissue viability and has worked with podiatrists. She makes the comment that there sometimes lacks common consensus around treatments and this fosters missed opportunities. Dr Fania Pagnameta points out in a similar vein putting podiatrists on the vascular ward produced incredible results (Podiatry Now, 2020).

Tarr (Landscape interview 2020) embraces this within his own diabetic department emphasises how important offloading is to help patients from re-ulcerating. This same message is extended by Tahira Bashir a dietician who works with podiatrists within a multidisciplinary team (MDT).

Head of Podiatry in Harrogate & District NHS Foundation Trust, Robin Hull, extols the MDT approach to rheumatology working within MSK services.

All of these examples have been taken from a recent publication by the College of Podiatry and demonstrate how patches of podiatry have had exemplary recognition from fellow professionals, but core podiatry and the wider function of podiatry is still misunderstood. Hull says that; *'after 38 years as a podiatrist, I still spend time explaining what podiatry is.'*

PODIATRY IS A MEDICAL SUBJECT

BoFAS[8] tells the public that chiropodists,

> While they study some general medical principles, they have not been trained in the diagnosis and treatment of general medical and surgical conditions.

What has not been said is that podiatrists are medically trained, but that they are not medically qualified. For some reason this is forgotten and yet it is no small point. When I asked BoFAS administrator Jo Millard the following question in July 2018

> How many orthopaedic surgeons are currently practicing foot surgeons? On an earlier site this was 400, does this remain about the case?

> I am afraid that we don't have results for your question as not all practicing foot & ankle

---

[8] British Orthopaedic Foot & Ankle Society formed 1983 as part of an interest group associated with the British Orthopaedic Association.

surgeons are members of our society. Regards
Miss Jo Millard BOFAS Administrator.

It was *estimated* by this author that there were about
700 joint dedicated UK foot surgeons in and around
2017-18 between the different professions, BoFAS,
CoP and IOCP.

How is information communicated?

Apart from professional attitudes, the information
provided can come in the form of a 'Question &
Answer' format. Short posts on websites, referring
to the above organisations, form majority of the
information delivery.

OSGO, an independent podiatry group offering
services to members uses a title curiously derived
from Osgood-Schlaater disease and is another
welcome competitor in the field for promoting
podiatric health care in the UK. OSGO deals with
their members and not the public, and provides a
wide range of information leaflets that can be
purchased, but differs little from the College or
IOCP where leaflets for patients can be purchased
by members to give to the public. Such information
re-enforces management planning and options, as
well as dealing with risks and benefits from such
interventions. This does not account for custom
leaflets by individuals.

The NHS relies on its own web based information
and NHS departments also develop their own

product ranges. The drive to genericise information however can be erroneous because different practises may exist and anything that speaks of protocol can be broken with unintended consequences.

This chapter does not seek to undertake a full analysis of each website and the quality of material therein. Any interested party accessing an open website will spend under a minute, in some cases <30 secs, deciding if the site is appropriate. Sites do change to meet new demands and readers can make their own decisions. The use of visual media is limited to one aforementioned site which promotes its activities in film. The three sites do not have any sound bites, which are short passages to say what they stand for. The correction however might come from BoFAS, where a certain amount of narrative is explaining why they, orthopaedics, are different to chiropodists[9] (sic).

How do patients get to podiatrists?

The larger percentage of patient referrals still come from general medical practitioners who have different views as to how to use podiatrists. Even

---

[9] The views held by BoFAS are affected by their general opposition to podiatrists practising foot surgery as non-medics. This has been exemplified during the noughties in newspapers such as The Daily Mail and The Telegraph. The issue over title has long been a cause for disagreement while the Faculty of Podiatry of the College of Podiatry advises the use of 'podiatric' as a prefix to 'surgeon' to make clear the distinction between types of surgeon.

NHS-111 direct defers to GPs about foot management in the first case. Putting in a search query on the foot is as likely to bring up the subject of diabetes rather than anything else (evidence June 2019). Many patients have prior knowledge and know foot = podiatrist but this is not always the case and many members of the public would not know the extent of scope of the profession.

Barriers to change become an academic topic and it is for the clinician to interpret scientific data. The term scientific has specific connotations in that it reveals evidence under controlled conditions. Randomness and ensuring spurious errors do not skew data is the aim of all researchers. Inferences as to why podiatry is not successful compared to other professions seems to come down to defining the limits of practice and how that scope is achieved.

On a one to one basis, or through village hall style talks, most members can leave a positive impact. Where sport is involved, dealing with groups of active men and women can escalate the local prestige of a practitioner's motivation to manage specific conditions and alter perceptions.

What has career image to do with promoting podiatry?

In reality the relationship between the brand and your service has a bearing on the ease and acceptance within healthcare models. The image behind a brand starts much earlier than we think.

The attraction to nursing or dentistry appeals to a certain type of person. The financial driver is important to many, to others it is the idea of caring for people. Experience in childhood and perceptions from parental influence and schools can make a difference. Labelling the value of a service to an extent that by the time we are adult and need to use a service dominates decision making. We will have a pre-conceived idea as to what that service offers and when to use it. If careers are a way to increase such recognition, then it is important that we use any mechanism at our disposal to increase positive publicity. A successful career structure is one way to achieve this. Certainly public relations, media, websites and hard information are vital, but they can only support a profession that desires change. Self esteem is often quoted in some questionnaire driven articles on what the profession and others think. Katie Noakes (2015) wrote a piece about professions that do not attract career interest;

> Podiatry is a lucrative yet somewhat unappealing job that is often overlooked by people when they are choosing a career. You would be dealing with tasks such as ingrown toenails, bunions, ulcers and many enthralling toe tasks and other fun-filled feet factors. Average earning of up to £29,000 per year are typical starting points for podiatrists and can ultimately increase up to £40,000, with the right experience and specialised training.

Even Noakes would be surprised by the College of Podiatry's latest published figures on earnings. Her figures may well relate to the NHS, but specialist podiatrists are able to enjoy salaries above £40,000 and in the independent sector over £100,000 depending upon the type of practice and and how many hours are worked. One of the big attractions of podiatry is that it is possible to work part-time or full-time while enjoying a good salary.

Perhaps Noakes could have written a different piece?

Podiatry is a profession with a good career structure and pay scale often overlooked by people when choosing a career. The role is integrated with many other health professionals as well as leading in foot health science. Because podiatrists are medically trained they are able to offer many services that maintain the nations foot health and mobility. Dealing with pain and discomfort is their primary aim, by managing deformity and skin integrity. These are vital ingredients for safe walking and restoring social integration. Maintaining the nation's health cannot be achieved without healthy feet (Author).

Does this put podiatry up there with embalmists?

Perhaps it is time to marry academic and straight talking narrative together. There is little point in relying on academic articles as the prime fascie point of contact. It is our role as academic clinicians to extract and interpret data for the purposes of our patients. Good media takes the best brands hopefully without distorting the truth. Nonetheless when we review what has been written, much should be re-written or rejected.

Getting Information Right

We should welcome Harrison-Blount's latest paper. It is important and for those that actually read the narrative will find it stretches the boundaries of thought. If we are to change, we need to focus on a simple message. We are a profession that manages mobility and deal with the foot, ankle and associated structures. To deal with the foot alone limits opportunities of the key bone structure that links the lower limb to the rest of the body. Some podiatrists have taken the bull by the horns and increased their scope outside of podiatry. *Is there anything wrong with this?* Surely changing scope is what we have been doing ever since the Council for the Professions Supplementary to Medicine was established in 1960, nearly a quarter of a century ahead of the HCPC.

The key elements of our work must be to manage pain, deal with the effects and consequences of deformity and preserve tissue within the foot and leg. In achieving each of these objectives we can maintain mobility.

Health starts with the foot!

We must make others believe there is one profession who can lead or we will continue to have other professions dictating our future.

5. Optimising Information through image

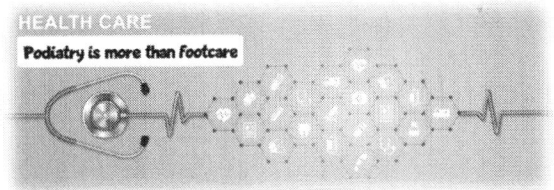

HEALTH CARE
Podiatry is more than footcare

Shutterstock/Birthpix

You need to optimise the use of information as a give-away product. This reflects your practice and of course promotes your specialty.

FACT SHEETS VERSUS GENERAL INFORMATION

When we set out to convert information we can do so by way of creating factsheets. Fact sheets provide data, hard statistics, and values to relate to, while information sheets may include facts and broader descriptions. In reality, it is difficult to write about every single treatment and so clinically we do our best to provide the most accurate impression of expectations.

Patient journeys were added to my own practice literature. Patients telling their story is powerful in a way that no clinician can represent. There is a balance between downplaying risks and impact against the benefits of success and treading a narrow pathway when providing information. Patient decisions are now made based on an ever growing task of complexity. Today it is the patient who must decide what pathway to travel and as clinicians, we must avoid being over persuasive. The bulk of information should be provided in advance of treatment and it is important for all of us, patients and clinicians to ensure those risks, no matter how small are included. As far as marketing your brand is concerned, it is important to divide information into bite size chunks. Promote key features and have material you can expand on. The use of short video pieces can be valuable and technological developments makes this ever easier and within the reach of most. I would however like to make a distinction between *factsheets* and *general information*. Take travel as an example.

<u>You want to travel from Birmingham to London</u>

<u>Facts</u> about that journey include *the time it takes, cost, services available en route, the speed of the vehicle, and options such as first or second class.*

These are all fixed, known details, although might have variables or ranges; e.g. *95 – 120 minutes travel time*.

General information will provide you with how you might get there with some options and perhaps could include the dos and don'ts associated with travel, how to connect to the internet once you are on the train and might even consider the type of food and drinks available. Alternative choices might include road travel, flight as well as train. Most likely the general information will include some of the facts and so the material could broaden.

Selected information

Specific information might be used, for example, one person might use a particular type of treatment where others do not. Information is governed by the limitations of individual practice experience and past results associated with what works well.

Dialogue is still important

Fact sheets cannot tell the whole story but they provide a taster. They do not represent choices alone. Factsheets do not always tell you about alternative treatment. Can you make a decision to proceed to a particular form of foot treatment? In accordance with current legal views, it is important to have the information explained so that dialogue exists. Reading the information and returning to a clinical office to go through those points is better than written information alone. A patient should be encouraged to return to the clinic before interventions to ensure all is understood. I have always encouraged my patients to write down their queries to avoid forgetfulness. Of course, minor interventions do not always require much preamble. In this case, choices would be limited, risks and impact minimal and the overall understanding would have less complexity. Examples might include injections to dull pain or simple remedial toenail management, the latter not requiring an analgesic injection.

What should you ask from a fact sheet?

Factsheets should be well written, have few spelling mistakes, be easy to read, laid out well and ideally not photocopied to death. Well presented factsheets mean the clinician cares as much about you as he/she does about the information they offer. This book is about selling and it is worth ensuring that photocopied material is best copy, but printing on demand is affordable. Make sure your essential information is printed. This makes sense as it truly reflects a positive image.

YOUR BASIC TOOLKIT

This should help drive your understanding of the consultation better. The factsheet will offer information about your care to help your patient make a choice and give them 'breathing room' for decision making. Having participated as a patient as well as a clinician I understand *what I want* and *what I need.*

As education has played an important role in extending our understanding of sciences, television has played host to horror stories and unsavoury conditions, and so we expect more for our investment. *"I'll leave it to you as you're the expert"* is no longer acceptable, the patient says, adding naively - *"You are the expert."*

As a former consultant, I used to cringe at this inaccurately held belief of me being an expert, not least because I was often the last resort for foot pain and many good people had already tried their best. But, as a professional I had to instill confidence.

Feedback

The precious time-period shared with your patient requires an aid-memoire to take away and this is where the factsheet comes in. So it acts as an aid to cover those parts of the consultation that need highlighting, things the patient needs to know and can be provoked to ask questions. The responses advise the provider with acknowledgement that something has been heard, understood and analysed. In many ways we need to be assured of all three aspects of this feedback. The factsheet does not replace the requirement for the clinician to explain the content of a factsheet. Your factsheet should provide useful data that can be used to make a decision. It fills in gaps. It should help patients consider priority.

What a Fact Sheet Does Not Do

Inevitably, factsheets do not answer all questions. This is simply because everyone has different views and a small percentage of patients will decline any desire for detail. There is nothing wrong with this until you need to make a decision that has a critical outcome that could leave the patient worse off afterwards. Drift to the internet and 'search' for information and you will find plenty, although most foot health information still comes from North American - USA sources. Again, there is nothing wrong with this as there is plenty of material but does it translate? There is no one reliable system so this is why I wrote my first book, 'Morton's neuroma' to fill in the gaps. Given so many aspects about the management of this condition and others it would be difficult to cover all in detail but I found a compromise in focusing on the top five.

The Patient Journey

The Patient Journey is unique and some patients write about their own experience in considerable detail. The day to day, even hour to hour, step by step description of human routine brings life into full colour, expanding on the shades of those realities that can fill many with dread. Harnessing a story with the facts and analysing the stages is important. In some ways publishing a diary where everything went so well is not as helpful as one might think. We know from published information that not all treatment pathways as we call the journey are garnered with smooth travel. While I am a great fan of factsheets, patients rely on the clinician's advice and any other information offered, the more personal and tailored the better. If you are like me and devour information with relish, there comes a point when only the patient can make the final decision.

The reason that factsheets cannot provide all information is that for the most part they cover information from many sources. When in clinical practice my factsheets were pooled from over 100 centres and in this case, covered several thousand patient feedback reports based on the data held by my professional body. The other problem with factsheets is that once material runs to many pages of typed lines it is easy to put aside for another day.

Design

Headings help guide you to the right place. Multiple sheets (probably more than 5) require an index to guide the reader. The modern use of hyperlinking is wonderful but cannot work with a typed sheet or if a portable digital file (PDF) has been used as this tends to knock out the links.

Good Factsheets Follow Good Consultations

A good factsheet tells you something about the condition and how it arrived, that is unless you fell over and that swollen foot is now the obvious result of you acting less sincerely toward your own safety. I will call this knowledge; what, why, how...? and your instructional headings might be considered around such questions. A Q&A approach of pooled common questions is another valuable tool.

 A patient will want to know how will treatment impact on their life and for how long? Can I go back to work - or even, *should I go to work*? And *can I go on holiday, go dancing, go to the theatre and can I cope if I am on my own, and will it get worse?*

If you are an adult you have responsibilities if you have a family, or you are needed as a core member of the household as a carer. These factors may impact on your life so that prior knowledge is important before embarking on a treatment plan.

Is there something I can do to help myself? Is it practical to fix the problem myself? Do I take medication or have something provided to help me get around - different shoe, stick, dressing, removable appliance?

Treatment

Do nothing, do something, rest? Use medication (pain and anti-inflammatories), sort out an infection, apply dressings or splinting, buzzy electronic treatments (ultrasound or extracorporeal treatment), add heat or cold, perform an injection (sometimes steroids) or carry out some type of procedure we call invasive and might mean surgery. Developing treatment and designing therapy around your patient's need should always become the main driver for your business.

Investigations

The foot is part of the skeleton also known as the musculoskeletal system (bones and joints, muscles and ligaments). Does the patient need an investigation? X-ray, blood examination, urine and so forth, this can be used as part of your scope of practice bringing in all the elements that make up overall care. Make investigations part of your promotional delivery as this takes podiatry away from the non medical side of the image.

PROMOTE MORE THAN PODIATRY

Does the patient have a choice? Make sure they know what they have to pay, or want to pay and how much is it? That bit won't be in a factsheet but it should be available as it is now a condition of independent health provision. No patient should enter into any contract to investigate or have treatment without knowing the cost.

Podiatry does not just mean feet!

The NHS of course in the UK does not require any direct payment for treatment. Additional information that might follow on includes where other support can be found. Some of these related health areas include smoking cessation, loss of weight and dietary control. Making use of your medical knowledge screening for blood pressure abnormalities, and if you have the skill, heart sounds and pulse irregularities may need flagging to medically qualified professionals. These key points may not be regarded as part of podiatry but failure to realise the value of first line provider skills which most podiatry practices could offer is an abrogation of ability.

For example:

- Habits smoking and alcohol
- Weight (BMI >35)
- Blood glucose abnormalities
- Cardiac signs of disease including claudication
- Peripheral neuropathy
- Analgesic drug overuse
- Signs of depression
- Skin lesions of concern
- Self-harming and domestic / child abuse

Some of the features above may require additional course development, but whatever you do as far as continuous professional development is concerned, do make sure you optimise on the value of promotion. **Podiatry is not just feet**!

USING INFORMATION TO OPTIMISE YOUR BRAND

There are several ways you may promote foot health care. Use your logo (see chapter 9) wherever and whenever you can to announce your presence.

Date and place your location on all your published materials. This might comprise a labelled drawing highlighting key facts. List choices and emphasise any risks. Tear off pads can be made up for nominal costs. Or, generate the picture electronically. Where you use anything printed promote your identity.

A leaflet will provide the patient with a list of information offering a concise summary of key elements they need to know. A professionally produced leaflet is powerful and can be passed between patients, their friends and family reflecting an image of your business, product and brand.

Some organisations publish booklets which are A5 stapled information with eight pages or more. Others may even have published books, although most do not have a large market or funding unless you are organisations of magnitude such as the

British Diabetic Association which has a bookshop. A quick look at their booklist does not just emphasise the disease but looks at diet. Once food becomes the subject, the parallel offshoots are endless as healthy cooking and life styles resonate with a broader readership. This latter angle is something podiatrists in the UK do not optimise. There are plenty of parallels where foot disease and good health can be partnered.

In my series of electronic factsheets launched from my website, I have used video film as 'YouTube' and made some films for a little longer than 5 minutes. You can see my example associated with making a bunion pad at www.consultingfootpain.co.uk. Considerations for producing video do need to include sound, lighting and editing out unwanted material. Using smart phones and tablets are fine for short bursts.

Hyperlinking information using external sources is both popular and effective. Newsletters and information delivered by electronic mail allows a large amount of information to fit into a smaller space and remain obscured until required. While this is the way forward be mindful of your individual patient's ability and preference. Having mentioned video, I should add Podcasts that use recorded voice. This has been an education resource for many years but there are serious opportunities often freely accessible with products such as *Podbean.*

6: The Burden of Foot Health

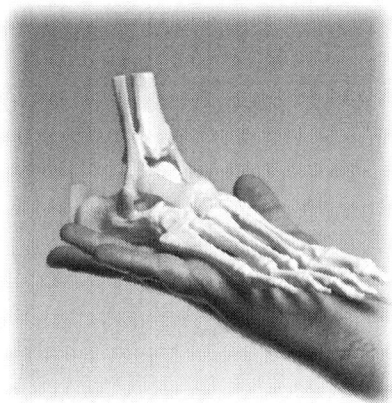

Shutterstock/Bart Sadowski

Although this chapter is called burden of foot health, the burden of care has parallel lines and associations with all aspects of health. In their paper O'Neill and Ross (2009) state within their abstract;

Burden of care is a concept emerging in the literature that describes the physical, emotional, social, and financial problems that can be experienced by family caregivers. This concept may be useful to heighten understanding of the family caregiving experience and as such may provide a framework for nursing practice and research[10].

There is a balance between each of these four underline paradigms and evidence which supports what we as podiatrists should deliver. In 2019 I penned an article called *'We should always have an opportunity to change attitudes'* where the emphasis of our brand related to the image of podiatry. So how should we package podiatry and why should we go along with the need for burden of care?

NHS REFERRAL PATTERNS

Most podiatrists do not see the NHS as a business but as an 'employer' for their skills. However, one Chief Executive said to me of my own efforts to push boundaries, *'David. without people like you we would never progress!'* Kind words although the effort required to bring change was exhausting.

When looking at quantitative findings Bowen and Edwards (2019) reported that 3% of of GP encounters related to foot pain in some way of which just over half a million (567,000) was associated with foot and ankle pain.

Fifty-five percent were female against 45% male. Upon further analysis, of 346,000 patients, most were referred to orthopaedics or physiotherapy with

[10] O'Neill's paper was reproduced in 2011 in Health Care Women although originally published in 2009.

50% going to podiatry and nursing. This caused the team some concern when they were investigating why rheumatological foot complaints had less priority than diabetic foot complaints. Both these conditions tend not to be managed in the type of numbers in the independent sector as they do in the NHS.

Pointing to a Useful Brand

The area of podiatry 'At Risk' conveys impact that we can build on. While this translates into diabetes for most, the erudite and wise realise this can expand into any condition that puts limb and life in jeopardy.

Language changes as the understanding of a subject becomes clearer. The brand of biomechanics led to sports podiatry which today has more substantive post-graduate education through a range of formal courses. All so often a title assumes a mantel only later to be identified as a smaller cog in the engine room. We will meet this later in the guise of orthotics (orthoses), diagnostic hand held Doppler and local anaesthetic as living examples of change.

Diabetic specialism

The specialism of diabetes was perhaps the first and most significant area to breakthrough the barrier of core podiatry image. Why? It captured the belief that a real cost saving could be achieved. Cost savings lubricate the moving components of logic. To those focused, conservative management would lead to salvaging limbs that otherwise might be lost to amputation. The associated savings by minimising hospitalisation were the very objective of this new brand.

Podiatric Surgery

Another specialty that rocketed to recognition was podiatric surgery. This has now expanded into the field of the 'at risk foot'. While diabetic care and podiatry required fewer battles than podiatric surgery, it came down to competition in the end. What was helpful and valued by one specialty was to another an anathema.

Rheumatology

'At risk' resonates as a career label and brand. Loss of limb versus saving a limb, keeping people functional starts to appeal to reason and common sense. A little behind diabetes, came podiatry and the arthritic foot focusing initially on rheumatoid disease. In fact, this was my first specialism in 1979 as I buddied up to the rheumatology service at our General Hospital. Rheumatology is more than just joints, it is all connective tissue overlaid with immunology and genetics, encompassing the at risk foot and tissue management.

The question raised by recent research has sought to answer why rheumatology is not as successful as the publicity around NHS diabetic footcare.

If the *physical, emotional, social, and financial* problems associated with diabetes is so well considered why not rheumatology? And we are not talking about rheumatoid arthritis as a single entity.

Funded by the National Institute for Health & Research, Professor Cathy Bowen's team looked at reasons for variations in referral pattern (2019). Endorsed by the College of Podiatry and Arthritis and Musculoskeletal Alliance (ARMA), they set out not just to crunch data but to seek answers. This meant asking the stakeholders, the GPs and commissioners who understood what podiatry was but did not understand the scope. As with the business side of the independent sector much comes down to finance, cost and efficiency. Bowen goes on to explain in a webinar much of the methodology behind the project and available on YouTube.

Why were foot pain patients referred to orthopaedics?

Bowen considers the acute sector is easier to access than the community sector where in the case of the latter the pathways are more complicated. She considers that podiatry often has a '*muddy pathway*'. It is easier to refer into a diabetic set up, or MSK, rather than for non-diabetic foot care. The systems have been better developed alongside multi-disciplinary teams often linked with other professionals such as physiotherapy. Triaging for surgery became very successful in my own experience. Patients could either go to orthopaedics or podiatric surgery in the NHS. This worked as we had a protocol in place and all the GP had to do was refer into one gateway of care and the rest followed.

> It is much better now that we have a central point of management and we can see patients within days. Tarr[11]

The relationship Tarr has with his local orthopaedic department, as an extended scope (diabetes) podiatrist, also clarifies why his work is so well supported in the NHS, not least as he works with general surgeons who specialise in vascular work. Furthermore, Tarr believes you don't need as many podiatrists in a team because working with GP and ward nurses act as a screen and flexible referral. Tarr's experience is not one of an isolated example in the UK. Frameworks and standards of care exist in abundance when compared to arthritis. Bowen certainly believes that until more evidence is gathered and housed within the repository of evidence by the National Institute for Health Care and Excellence (NICE), that creating the same provision for podiatry with arthritis, as with diabetes, will fail to be optimised. However, she is encouraged that scientific evidence is growing.

[11] Ian Tarr, extended scope podiatrist in diabetic care at Walsall NHS Trust provided a landscape interview on setting up his diabetic service April 2020

Simple Communication

We should never turn away from underpinning podiatry with academic evidence despite the suggestion that too much academic discussion can fail to achieve the message. But, the active face of podiatry is a business and hopefully we can agree on this. Our job as clinicians is as much about translating and transposing information as it is to provide treatment for patients. *Transposing* is used in the musical sense trying to take one set of notes and changing the key so that the sound alters. Consider an explanation given to a patient thus;

> Your foot pain is due to pronatory forces caused by your inability during midstance to counter postural instability, or that corns are due to biomechanical irregularity

It is doubtful that anyone would suggest this line of explanation to a patient, anymore than someone would suggest that inflammation is due to an over reaction to mast cell interaction, serotonin release or T-cell mediation. Equally on the converse side of the argument do we benefit from highlighting that a toe nail pierces the flesh as in IGTN? (Tollafield 2019), or that the most common cause of heel pain is due to plantar fasciitis when the 'ligament' running under the heel becomes swollen. Perhaps we must ask ourselves, what is true, what is accurate and what is acceptable for public understanding of the complexity of foot pathology?

When should a Patient Seek Help?

Language is important and so is the message that podiatry can help positively. That we will advise you on the best treatment, or that if your foot problem is not improving then you should seek the help of a podiatrist. One organisation suggests that 3 weeks of a foot condition is *when* to seek help. I am unsure I would wish to make such a blanket statement about a specific time because some conditions need earlier attention and in truth podiatry does not routinely offer or publicise an emergency service. There are aspirations as to what we would like to do and represent, versus what we actually can do and achieve in practice. A professional body might give the impression of delivering a specific service or skill, but it may well be that only a smaller percentage can convert those aspirations into an active service.

Traditional Podiatry

Brand podiatry sits alongside an image of routine. Styled as repetitive care allied to managing key elements as in nails, corns, flat feet, ingrowing toe nails, verrucae. Maybe a bunion or hammer toe might appear in the equation, but do we cure these? The loyal patient who returns regularly may feel well served and promote the service. As we will see in a later chapter this can be used as testimonial. A data base[12]shows the most frequent five diagnoses and shown in descending order from most to least as:

- Hallux valgus
- Hammer toes
- Hallux rigidus
- Morton's neuroma
- Onychocryptosis

Clearly if the lay public were to read this we would state, *bunion*, bent or *deformed toe, stiff/arthritic* type big toe, *nerve entrapment* and *ingrown toe nail*. Use of complex language needs to be tempered to fit the audience. The data base statistics is biased toward foot surgery and podiatric surgeons who receive such referrals (from GPs) can reflect on these common diagnoses. At the time of writing the PASCOM-10 database runs to over 135,000 patients and shows 81,000 recorded consultations from 139 centres.

Because general podiatry does not populate this database, and where it does it does so only in small numbers, the diagnoses might be different. We lean on other sources for general podiatry. For podiatrists and maybe others, the **Top-10**

---

[12] Data accessed 08/04/20 PASCOM-10 database College of Podiatry. Ten years of data taken between 1 Jan. 2010 to 8 April 2020

breakdown diagnoses is interesting where hallux valgus represents 30%, hammer toes 23%, hallux rigidus drops to 11.2%, Morton's neuroma 5.7%. Thereafter ingrown toe nails (5.4%).

Other conditions were represented by less than 2%. Fasciitis and flat foot fall below this at 1.7% and 0.4% respectively. It is of course more likely that corns are referred to podiatrists rather than podiatric surgeons (1.6%) but other data acquired suggests presenting problems included

- Arthritis in feet
- Tailor Bunion
- Ganglion
- Heel pain
- Corns

Core Podiatry

Having met many podiatrists who have no desire to undertake surgery, and why should they? I was impressed that a number had developed strategies that involved different approaches to podiatric delivery of care. The podiatrist who loves home visits is one engaged in realising the social importance as much as the support that podiatry bestows elsewhere. Farndon (2006) has coined the term Core Podiatry and this is a useful because it encapsulates the basis upon which British podiatry developed from chiropody. Specialism in podiatry however has become important to recruits from the eighties and beyond and possibly no less so for the advent of advanced courses including degrees and diplomas. The more specialised we become the easier it is to drift from the core elements of the practical aspects taught when first entering professional training. The patient who seeks a quick solution will be disappointed if they do not achieve resolution. The problem with podiatry is that many conditions are not cured and can at best be supported. We have called this *palliation* and this must be re-branded.

Farndon (2009), researching the subject of epidemiology has reviewed the type of common work carried out by generalists, those podiatrists that deliver the bulk of foot care to the nation either in the independent sector or NHS.

> A summary of combined surveys found that between 20–78% of people suffer from corns, callus and bunions, between 20–49% have lesser toe deformities and 28–56% have toenail problems.

Core podiatry involves treatment of the nails, corns and callus and also giving footwear and foot health advice. From a cohort of 1047 patient questionnaires 75% of patients (26-95 years) had podiatric problems.

Management of the pain elements of core podiatry can be sustained or improved in 75% of cases using simple outcome measures such as visual pain scores. In their database podiatric surgeons suggest that corns fall to below 2% diagnostic reasons for referral and forms the 10th most common condition referred. Farndon (2015) identified corns and callus in 26% cases resulting in management of similar conditions in 19% of cases in a typical working day.

Providing accurate data is a challenge but data is powerful once we reach high numbers. The delivery of core support as a service is important, but for some it is easy to disassociate oneself from routine features of podiatry but why? It is at this point one feels it is important to reflect.

> After 18 months following qualification I felt frustrated that I could not cure patients and so inevitably this led me toward podiatric surgery. I realised that it was not the fact that I could not cure as much as I did not understand why I could not cure?

ALTERING THE DIRECTION OF YOUR SERVICE

Historically the profession delivered core podiatry and because this has been seen to be less attractive to the very people who deliver this necessary care, internally our own profession allowed core podiatry to diminish and be seen as boring and too routine. And yet it is vital. Routine practice encapsulated by maintenance care drove many to seek a different approach, often depending on orthotic strategies.

However, funded research that has been carried out is dominated by diabetic and rheumatological care rather than research into the routine of core podiatry in majority of cases. It is important to reflect that this service is not only essential but it is unique in respect of debridement skills. All professions have repetitious duties. Podiatry is no different. I was certainly a typical podiatrist who bent my manager's arm to undertake nail surgery, at the time represented by a fraction of podiatrists. By 1978, biomechanics was branded by US podiatrists as the new way forward. This diverted podiatry toward an orthotic revolution that gave many the impression all matters foot health could be solved with contoured plastic. Although inappropriately named today the subject assumes the latest version, MSK science, based on kinesiology and kinematics. Some balance has to redress over subscription of the so called *prescription orthotic.* Modular orthoses offer similar value to the now older casted methods. Perhaps it was inevitable that sub specialisms emerged. 'Verruca specialist' and 'nail surgery specialist' established themselves because these were break away subjects formerly divorcing themselves with the drudgery of *'cut and come again'* . A term equally repulsive to most podiatrists because of the strong relationship with *pedicure*. This had nothing to do with the action itself which could be immensely satisfying once a diseased nail was cut back, the nail bed dressed and healed, restoring comfort and averting further complications.

Debridement

In 1983 I was sent to a hospital by my boss. Working out of a room without windows, the elderly patients were brought down to a room no better described as a 'cupboard'.

Upon examining the foot with an angle poise light I could see a lesion that hid potential breakdown.

'Don't touch that,' the nurse said, *'the doctor insists that this is left alone because of his concern that this could be something bad!'*

Firstly, the ward doctor was wrong, and secondly, my skill was not recognised, save for the fact that podiatry was a feature available to the hospital's geriatric population. Being a person who can see someone else's error and having complete confidence in my podiatric education and skills, the blackened tissue was removed to allow healthy new skin to be exposed and heal. I recall the nurse being somewhat impressed. A sharp knife, no anaesthetic and no bleeding. *Show don't tell!*

> So how does a podiatrist know that the black
> skin was not dry gangrene, and when to debride?
> Is this not worthy of promotion?

The public in some cases see areas of debridement as representative of activities linked to traditional pedicure because we allowed them to see this as pedicure. Our US counterparts rebranded footcare as a medical sub-specialty. In reality we failed to see a brand opportunity in routine (core) care.

Economic Factors

Unfortunately, there are some activities in the field of private practice where limitations are imposed. This might relate to a patient being unable to have optimum care due to cost. Establishing a practice such as podo-paediatrics requires specialised staff for invasive management in some healthcare settings.

Podo-paediatrics

Paediatric podiatry would emerge encapsulating all aspects of childhood foot health. Whether one believes that paediatrics should have a specialty will depend on scope and future development within the health service, which is unlikely. Safe guarding children now plays a major role in who are able to deal with children. Some hospitals limit podiatric surgery for patients over 16 years of age unless a specialist children's nurse is available. The staffing costs can play a major part in running some services based on specialised staffing. The role of general podiatry in managing diabetes and arthritis can be affected by chronic disease, poor finance and home support. This is where the NHS tend to come into their own as providers.

Patients with higher risk conditions still manage to buy insured support whether from the big private health care providers or by small hospital savings groups. Of these two groups, the latter often pays out for podiatry treatment while the larger providers pay for specific care pathways such as injections, surgery and in some cases for biomechanical assessments and gait analysis.

Orthotic and Footwear Provision

At college we spent hours gluing, heating and pressing thermoplastics onto plaster casts, but this skill was soon to diminish. The study of prosthetics and orthotics is now hi-tec and the use of third party laboratories makes sense. Growing awareness of COSHH[13] underpinned health and safety, but increased the cost of delivering orthotic services. This was another reason why NHS departments withdrew orthotic laboratory provision in many departments, favouring other services to provided footwear and insoles. Perhaps the exception to the rule was the diabetic departments like the one managed by Tarr who, in the NHS, bought in pre-made specialist footwear which was not only cheaper than bespoke footwear, but more effective, and less likely to end up at the bottom of a wardrobe.

---

[13] COSHH stands for Control of Substances Hazardous to Health and comes under the purview of the Health & Safety Executive (HSE)

Implementing all the safety features of an orthotic lab. has become more difficult to justify. The deployment of podiatrists in a workshop when patients need to be treated became less tenable and yet this was the career that some of us entered into. In a third world country this may be more applicable because of a need to use mixed skills.

The hours formerly used to develop psycho-motor skills such as 'core debridement' would diminish as degree courses had to re-apportion time to formal academic subjects. New skills and approaches to orthotic management emerged with the mass produced modalities from gel toe sleeves to ready made cheap inlays. Silicone moulds still remain in place alongside chair side appliances. As time passes it will be the older practitioners that retain these skills. The modern and younger podiatrist will be attracted to handing out well presented appliances. These will enhance the brand of podiatry and are instant deliveries as would be expected of an on-line service. Musculoskeletal kinesiology is too much of a mouthful to brand, but abbreviated to MSK does well. This nomenclature will inevitably re brand.

The Under-Rated Service

Footwear and deformity … these components of foot health either clash dramatically or create foot health harmony. Footwear crosses all aspects of podiatry. Advisory or educational foot health has suffered poor funding and lacks support and to some extent investment as a formal subject. In 1993 I met one such colleague in a trust who was the go--to-man for footwear advice. A vital subject that if understood held the key to serious promotional foothealth potential. When he passed away unexpectedly, and before his time, a yawning gap arose in our service. His post was not refilled! The reason? Footwear held little attraction for most in the department and for the Management; was this really something that added any value to treatment? After all it was invisible. Invisible activities that have little measurable benefit tend to sink to the bottom of the glass.

A regular feature existed in the former Society (of Chiropodists) journal during the eighties when Brian L Berry wrote enthusiastically about footwear. An attempt was made to take up the mantle but without passion and motivation this regular feature was subsumed by other material. Good quality articles (Williams, 2006) have been published but the momentum has not been sustained. Podiatrists as a profession have failed uniformly to associate themselves with the footwear industry. The approach has been more about tickling at the edges rather than immersion. Former associations with Clark's shoes in Street, Somerset, beloved by many students sadly ended in the last decade of the 20th century.

Most of us know the history of footwear development only too well but do we know of all the options available, material designs and their research potential? It was only when I had to teach footwear and engage with the research foundation called Shoe and Allied Trade Association (SATRA) at Kettering that I appreciated the potential for our then diploma course. To those with initiative this subject is long overdue recognition. This is partly because we talk about shoe advice but it is not formalised as a specialty, and partly because the need to remain up to date with footwear is not attractive. Footwear is a science and podiatry does not optimise its relationship with industry in the UK. Such inaction might well be losing out on a trick. In the private sector little if anything is published to demonstrate an opportunity for specialism unless one looks at the commercial world of outlets such as Shuropody and Scholl's that utilises podiatrists in a sales role.

In his NHS extended podiatry post in diabetes Tarr says of footwear provision;

> We would fix the foot then they (the patients) would go out and buy cheap shoes from the local market and re-ulcerate their foot. We are paying £30 a pair via the NHS. This means they don't need the orthotist's bespoke shoes. It saves masses of money but what's more they wear them whereas the orthotist's shoes cost £400-£500!

NHS Management and Teams

For the most part this chapter emphasises our relationships with the clinical side of podiatry. Management by podiatrists today is a rarer commodity compared to 4 decades ago when every aspiration was to be a manager of which a few mistakenly believed they were superior to their workforce. Today, managers may just as likely emerge from another profession, physiotherapy, speech therapy or nursing where departments are larger and where the drive is toward multidisciplinary teams (MDTs). While this regimen is more akin to the NHS, some work in the independent sector as MDTs with a different emphasis but similar outcome.

The word private was a word that became corrupted and equated to greed in the eyes of some. A strange reaction in a country with a democratic and capitalistic outlook. The independent sector currently makes up the bulk of podiatric practice activity. There is less managerial control, often better remuneration, and the scope offered can be wider than the ever growing constraints of the NHS.

The internal World Versus the Global Market

Does the outside world understand any of this? Probably not and in many ways the two sectors (NHS & Independent) focus on different aspects of foot health. So what do we learn from all this discussion and reflection between different activities? That there is a need to communicate clearly about our goals. Are podiatrists effective and which brand should we promote? Whether you are an NHS based practitioner or strictly in the independent sector, both groups can learn from common denominators. What we do need is to ensure that the internal market or the profession does not delude itself if it is to remain or even grab more of the global foothealth market. So we might ask, how are we going to do it?

7: Looking beyond the canvas

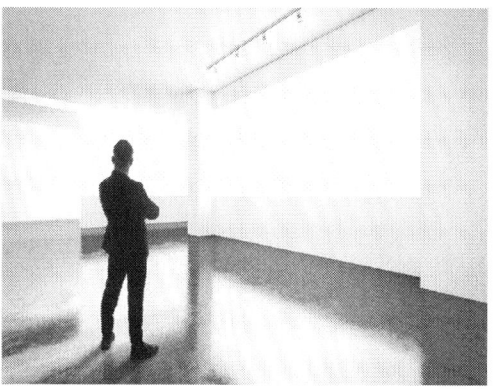

Shutterstock/Sfio Cracho

COMPETING

Upon graduating your method of competition moves from academic goals to your career as a podiatrist. If you work in the NHS, you might wish for promotion. In the independent sector you are competing for business by reputation. In the previous chapter I looked at the profession and its sub groups that have emerged over five decades.

The stark message is that nothing stays the same for ever. A need to constantly review one's own market is essential for survival. The regulation of podiatry still requires observation in regard to integrity when advertising and so you cannot say *'I am better than...'* Equally criticism of others, while tempting, often backfires on the unwise practitioner who believes they can achieve a jump on a colleague.

The NHS podiatric workforce has shrunk compared to other allied health professions and so there is a recruitment drive. New opportunities open up all the time, but the NHS has been enshrined in delivering to those most at risk. Does this minimise the opportunity to expand ideas and develop new services? We have to consider new ideas, not use emotional resentment.

When a colleague took an interest in biomechanics his manager was initially reluctant to allow him time to work with a bioengineer. The saving grace was that the podiatrist was introduced to the bioengineer by the manager. With not a little persuasion the podiatrist sought to undertake research through the bioengineer's department, which was part of the rheumatology unit. Seven months later, with two publications in the can the manager felt he had achieved something positive. The podiatrist had a life long friend in the bioengineer and new doors opened for both because of the collaborative association.

The moral of the Tale

New pathways of opportunity will never open unless we are prepared to take a risk and go with our heart. Three people benefitted, the podiatrist, the bioengineer and the manager.

Branding doesn't happen overnight, and certainly takes longer than many believe.

> Your brand is what other people say about you when you're not in the room. Jeff Bezos, Amazon

From birth to success, independent practice will take years because it will depend on competition, local community attitudes, your own focus on what your community wants or needs. Sometimes people do not know what they need and this is where podiatry can capitalise.

Sonia Gregory (Freshsparks) says,

> Building a brand is definitely a process. However, the ongoing effort will result in establishing long-term relationships with your customers. This can lead to a steady increase in word-of-mouth referrals, and advocacy for your service.

Is ability to brand determined by age?

Career podiatrists fall into an age bracket anywhere between 21 – 75+. The plus is added here to include older colleagues, although there will be fewer podiatrists in the plus age bracket. With extended employable years and a society intolerant to worship formal retirement age, there is no end point set in tablets of stone. For those within the younger age spectrum, social media and methods combining websites with Search Engine Optimisation (SEO) come more easily. The skills acquired involve blogging and promoting their views on the internet stage, often visually.

I attended a conference in 2018 and listened to one speaker talking about podiatry business. She spoke well, had motivation and enthusiasm, but also had an acute sense of awareness in the world of business. This quality is becoming more essential and for those who feel 'private practice' is a no-go area; think again. Think outside the box, prepare to change, consider that new skills can emerge from areas previously thought irrelevant. In this light the painting analogy starts to make sense. Stand back and reflect with new vision.

BASIC ADVERTISING

> You cannot brand if you don't understand what you are branding! Branding is generating awareness about your business using marketing strategies and campaigns with the goal of creating a unique and lasting image in the MARKETPLACE - Gregory

How do we see ourselves?

Podiatrists have public images that we ideally might not wish. Look at the image over the page. The podiatrist sits at the lowest end of the body, feet propped up on the woman's lap. But who thinks this is demeaning? Certainly not the patient, who is grateful to the podiatrist in serving a need that she cannot meet herself. The podiatrist on the other hand uses knowledge to provide a skill, identify sub-ungual damage and debrides any tissues.

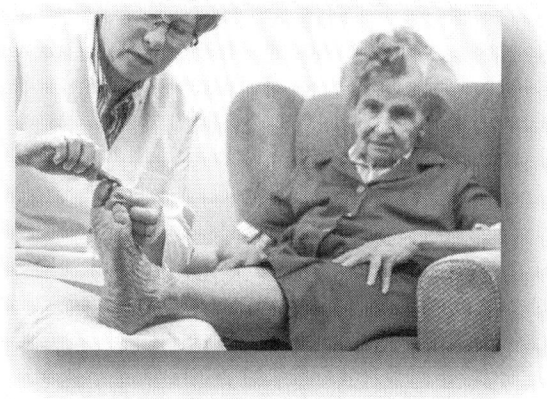

Shutterstock/ Alexander Raths

The use of a surgical instrument, professional nippers has to consider **method and prevention of cross infection**. A knowledge of microbiology and pathology is essential as a standard to meet care delivery. The point one must make is that podiatry is not about cosmetic nail care but assessing damage that if left could escalate. Shah-Hamilton (2020) makes this point even more clearly when it comes to patients with cancer. Many treatments can cause nail pathology and maintaining tissue care is paramount not least because patients may have diminished immunological support.

You can create great publicity using the media but if the message is unclear and does not hit the right market, the message and expenditure used to put the message together is lost. Branding comes down to message and how to promote that message. Here is the dilemma. How does a professional promote their?
image within the framework of regulation and professional ethics?

In 1980 the professional body and Council for Professions Supplementary to Medicine imposed advertising limits. The style, size and words used were rigidly enforced. Your professional sign and its layout also came under scrutiny. Six adverts were permissible in one local newspaper A neighbouring podiatrist working 4 miles away reported me for using the word podiatrist even though I had completed my qualification[14], then (MPodA) in 1981. This was a senior competitor trying to steel a jump on a less experienced member of the profession.

---

[14] At the time the title podiatrist was not used and only recognised by the Podiatry Association (see chapter 1). Having completed the requirements of one body the chiropodist concerned tried to stop my activities by using an underhand method by complaint and internal nepotism. This was not upheld by any party.

Reflection

The aforementioned tale exposes our moral judgement. Some will be respected while others will feel the weight of professional animosity.

By 1996 I had published two books for the profession. However, having set out the principles of podiatric surgery in one book (Tollafield, 1997), I thought little of this and in fact believed that I had suggested these same principles equally applied to all podiatry. Later these principles were put down to 4 aims, and yet erroneously considered within surgery (Tollafield, 2005). Having reviewed my original copy, I realised the folly of my beliefs. The original narrative had suggested pain, tissue preservation and deformity management were our aims. Today and in light of renewed thinking over our 'image' I now realise this all fits a mnemonic – M.A.I.D and in my various talks I have promoted this as a branding tool for our raison d'être.

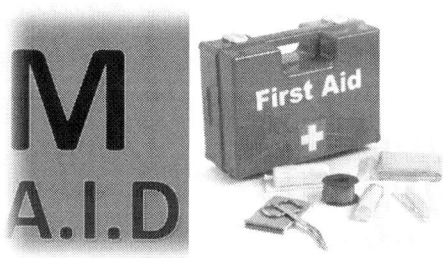

Tollafield-Shutterstock/zerbor

We Should Brand What We Do

Mobility (M) is the outcome of our effort. Patients who cannot mobilise lose their independence. Morbidity rises and health deteriorates with organ failure. Loss of independence adds to the burden. For the individual, this is equally damaging. Loss of income, the ability to care for family or self, and to engage with a normal society structure can lead to depression. Depression is a slow poison.

Alignment (A) is the management of deformity and stability. From lumps and bumps to flat feet, disruption of the midfoot, and negative influence upon the proximal limb.

Integrity (I) of tissue affects every level of the skeletal framework with a strong emphasis on softer tissues from skin (epidermis), dermis, fat, tendons, ligaments, blood and nerve networks to joints. The bulk of podiatry deals with epidermal-dermal changes. More often this concept is packaged under tissue viability.

Discomfort (D) relates to pain and is the driver that raises awareness that all is not well and there is a need to seek help where pain medication fails.

Let's analyse these four objectives

If pain is the driver, then the cause fits alignment and integrity. All three impact upon mobility. Fix these and the outcome will improve. Testing these concepts further, take Morton's neuroma or tibial nerve compression in the tarsal tunnel where we see pain as the prime symptom. However, it is the tissue that has deteriorated at neural level, probably due to alignment pathology (A) and as a result tissue has deteriorated and no longer functioning normally. Likewise, inflammation and infection are features

111

of tissue integrity. The need for the body to deal with either can release chemicals and cellular reaction destabilising tissue. While the necrotic ulcer is the type of feature that springs to mind, it is but one feature of tissue integrity. If the main foot tissues are at fault function alters with pain as a secondary feature. Each element will drive different responses but all will reduce mobility.

Who deals with the features of MAID?

The simple answer is that we all do. All podiatrists apply the concept of M.A.I.D. This is the reason behind our brand, to restore mobility by managing foot health optimally. This brand has taken ½ century to achieve and yet it always existed. A profession that once dealt with structures associated with skin and nails alone is inaccurate and yet it is still promulgated by some groups. Dictionary definitions are unhelpful and change across the English speaking world. A US based dictionary views a podiatrist differently to the British dictionary. Who sets the boundaries? Contrary to belief it is not the HCPC but the profession. Who is the profession? Well, it's us.

Self and Us

The key to branding is both self and us for we are stronger as a single image. Reflecting on the period up to and just beyond the State Registration Act 1960, which altered the direction of podiatry, we were driven into a corner that reflected a limited perspective of what we could do. Once it was the School, College and then later Universities that set boundaries, but in fact they only provided a basic platform for development. Progress thrived under the hands of groups prepared to stretch the boundaries.

If you were to look analytically at the two main podiatry organisations, the CoP and IOCP[15], both promote, regulate and stretch boundaries through their members, but in different ways. The HCPC, formerly the CPSM, only expects a baseline standard. Changes are in place to annotate the sub-specialty of podiatric surgery. While the HCPC does not interfere with scope, providing that there are checks and balances from the professions, the statutory body polices the registered podiatrist on behalf of the public.

---

[15] CoP College of Podiatry. IOCP Institute of Chiropodists & Podiatrists

REFLECTION ON TRADITIONAL MEDICINE

We see medicine like an amoeba having divided itself. First into physicians and surgeons where physicians were considered academically superior. From physicians and surgeons, they splintered into sub- groups. Doctors specialise then sub specialise, then if they enter modern day private practice, they specialise again within an already specialised field.

One of the attractive features of modern medicine, not without criticism, is the fact that a doctor today admits when a medical condition is outside his or her area. A recommendation for a referral would then be indicated. As a podiatric surgeon I worked within a medical framework in both the NHS and Independent sector. I was sent patients mainly with the elements of 'A' alignment allied to 'D' discomfort. Once I was found useful I had more referrals which then fell under 'I' tissue integrity. As time progressed, despite having a background in orthotic care, I no longer had the time to implement this area I had once excelled in. Furthermore, I was no longer at the top of my game to manage this side of podiatry. In fact, I started to realise that the medical profession was bypassing my own podiatry colleagues, who in some cases were dealing with *number problems* in the NHS. Even podiatrists were only too happy to shift patients into the surgical specialty. Of course this overloaded my service.

Distortion of a Brand

Surgery has a place but is not a panacea for all foot ails. As I now stand back from the coloured canvas on the wall, it is important to realise that podiatry can do so much more before surgery is considered. So obsessed was I in ensuring my specialty took on all aspects of foot health management, I failed to appreciate that we are only as strong as the sum of our parts.

Alien to refer?

The concept of referring on is still alien to some, and yet it does not damage reputation. One wonders why we do not share so readily? Is it loss of income from the practice? Or that there is no longer a regular rebooking? If that is the case, podiatrists are not doing their profession or patients justice. If as a podiatric surgeon I did well, my podiatry colleagues who referred patients were credited. If I did not perform well, my podiatry colleague was the fall back and I was regarded less. She would not be thought of any less for my failure.

The message is simple. We must work to our strengths and in working together control foot health delivery. We must know our limitations but collectively there is never a better time to reflect on our brand, which is based on what we actually do, and not wish we could do.

8: How do we deliver the message?

Shutterstock/Constantin Stancui

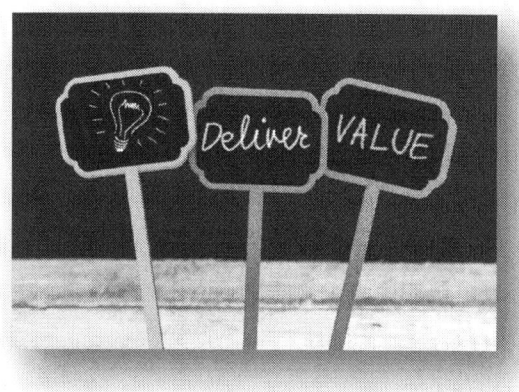

PUBLICITY

The modern era of fast communication and social media has both benefits and risks. Let's deal with the risk first and the cost to independent practice.

The cost of failed communication

The number one reason for a patient complaint arises from someone seeing no benefit from their consultation or treatment. Failure to communicate or respond to a patient can evoke annoyance. Delaying their appointment or keeping them waiting, although the lesser evil, falls into a common gripe. The net effect of any dispute can lead to the patient refusing to pay for their visit. This ultimately creates the knotty issue as to how to retrieve your consultation time fee.

> A colleague had referred a patient to me. The patient made an appointment and attended a booked consultation. After I had carried out a vascular assessment I pointed out that he needed to see a vascular surgeon. His circulation and ABI were clearly sub normal. He held out that I had not done anything for him. My time, expertise in confirming his problem and prognosis, let alone the need to refer to someone else, did not enter his head. The letter I wrote took time, required professional scribing and I had to pay for secretarial services.

Fee retrieval is a necessary evil, and signing up to agencies who will collect money for a fee, or going to small claims services[16] takes time out of a busy

---

[16] Collection services work on the basis of collecting your unpaid fee and taking a percentage cut once retrieved. The alternative method is to employ a small claims court system which is now achieved as an on-line service. A fee is payable and if liability is proven the fee will be reimbursed.

schedule. Naturally no-one wants to be in the position above but it provides a reflection of how important it is to be clear about why a referral is made. This was not my first experience. This does not help practice image, let along branding. You are left with two choices retrieve your money or write it off.

The best solution is to accept that this can happen and understand the patient's point of view. With every appointment make sure that communication is provided to make clear that consultations may not result in treatment and that advice is as much part of the skill being offered. You cannot demean your capacity by ignoring the fact that advice is still a billable component of the consultation. If comments are negative, think of a way of turning this around to positive

Dealing with poor feedback

If we deliver a positive message about podiatry, we must also provide assurances. If there is a money issue, deal with it. The solution. Act immediately. i.e as soon as you have an adverse response. If the reaction comes in through social media do not respond via social media, go to the patient directly. Face to face is best, but telephone at least followed by a letter summarising a) your understanding of the issue b) how you propose to deal with the concern c) actions that have been agreed. File a copy, date and time all correspondence.

BE POSITIVE. ALL FEEDBACK IS GOOD!

Admit if something has failed, not through negligence of course but through the process you took. *Show don't tell* how you have made it a valuable part of feedback. *Actions are greater than words alone.* This is not easy when you might feel that this was not your creation to start with. Never take it out on the patient. One of the failings of my own dentist on one occasion was when I could not confirm which tooth was hurting until he anaesthetised the wrong one. He was what we call *'old school'.* Some treatments should never dominate until required.

Website

Your website is an important tool for marketing your brand in this day and age.

> When you design your website: incorporate your voice, message, and personality into the content - Sonia Gregory.

She also says that profile pages for social media networks should be branded visually, and with your chosen voice for engagement. When it comes to social media I will let Sonia guide you (Gregory 2019). Refer to the reference section and guide to her website.

One podiatrist who signed-up to my Reflective Podiatric Practice RPP[17] is an avid vlogger and produced an A-Z on podiatry conditions. *How brilliant is that?* Observing a snap shot in terms of seconds, not minutes she could reach people on Facebook and Instagram. Video is a great medium but takes time. Your brand should be visible and reflected in everything that people see when looking at your business, product and service.

After leaving clinical practice I kept my website going but redesigned it into two components. Patient (*Footlocker*) and colleague-podiatrists (*Clinician Portal*). In fact, all my reflective articles come from Clinician Portal but they are not usually open access initially as I wanted to provide something that was unique for colleagues. Here is the point I have tried to make. If you have website, it will require time each month to keep updated. If it is basic it won't elevate you above your competitors. I spend hours updating my website as it is prime communication medium. Invest in someone to assist you if you do not have time, bearing in mind your job is to treat patients not spend hours writing material?

INFORMATION @ NHS & NICE

The National Health Service was established on 5th July 1948 and forms the backbone of Britain's

---

[17] RPP Reflective Podiatric Practice is published by Busypencilcase Communications Ltd (BPCC)

healthcare system. Its stands to reason then that statements about healthcare are backed by many authoritative sources, e.g N.I.C.E, the National Institute for HealthCare and Excellence. Established in February 1999, the first guideline ironically covered a flu product *Zanamir*. The first Public Health Guideline was published in March 2006 and thereafter NICE Care Pathways in May 2011. By 2012 75 pathways had been published. Bone and Joint conditions featured early.

So what do you publish? Moreover, where do we take information from? The most important ingredient when sharing information to promote is to stick to facts. If two independent sources agree then the facts are likely to be true, but they have to be truly independent. In chapter 4 much was covered on information and policies from the professional bodies. It is quite likely that some information is derived from the NHS website on health issues or from NICE. Of the two, the NHS carries the broadest information and many foot health conditions are created by different health Trusts via their local podiatry department. The information is patient friendly and has many inter-web links to other sites. The information on chilblains is one example of many given in the reference section.

NICE Pathways

NICE on the other hand looks at a limited range of treatments to establish their effectiveness through rigorous scientific peer review. Inevitably many of their pathways, although reviewed, are far from

current and the process takes a long time to complete based on quality randomised trials.

> NICE Pathways offer an easy-to-use, intuitive way of accessing a range of clinical, public health and social care information from NICE.
>
> They include up to date NICE guidance, quality standards and related information. ... NICE Pathways are for people who use NICE guidance. (NICE from the internet *accessed April 2020)*

If you establish a website and want to import information, both NHS and NICE sites are worthwhile. You can then back up any relevant material published by your preferred professional body. However, as a general recommendation the site called 'Footeducation' ranks high on the patient advisory reference scale (see panel).

Other web connections

At the time of writing there are a number of sites that will offer different foot health material. In the main these tend to have a surgical bias. However 'Footeducation.com' based in San Francisco has contributors from a wide panel of clinical experts and has built up a smorgasbord of information.

Physiotherapy sites often offer good information and individual orthopaedic sites are starting to deal with specific conditions. It seems that the professional organisations remain more loyal to the membership than to the broad public at this time.

ConsultingFootPain (CFP) is designed to cover common conditions with stories and a little research, mostly distilled down for the consumer. It mixes some material for clinicians at a more academic level but all material is available on-line. (www.consultingfootpain.co.uk). Public information is important and helps soften the swathe of hard sell.

What Should You Ask from a Factsheet, as seen on the next page and discussed in chapter 5 emphasises the importance behind design of a website articles.

The value of such an article is that it does not just stop at patients and lay readers but includes professionals, (Tollafield, 2019). The image over the page shows a sheet I designed for WordPress. The full article is accesses by selecting the panel shown to read more.

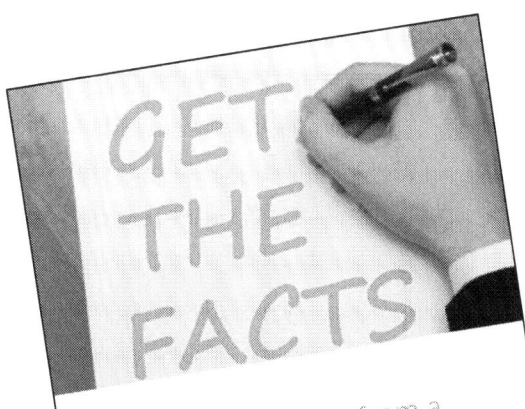

What should you ask from a factsheet?

by David Tollafield | Mar 23, 2020 | Clinician Portal, Factsheets and advice, Footlocker Hub, Publications | 0 Comments

What should you ask from a fact sheet?A Feature ArticleFactsheets should be well written, have few spelling mistakes, be easy to read, laid out well and ideally not photocopied to death. Well presented factsheets mean the clinician cares as...

read more

FootEducation is committed to helping educate patients about foot and ankle conditions by providing high quality, accurate, and easy to understand information.

In 2009, orthopedic foot and ankle surgeon, Dr Stephen Pinney recognized a need to provide quality patient-friendly education materials to ensure patients were well informed. Thus FootEducation was born.
Over the years, our commitment to providing high quality foot and ankle patient education has lead us to explore ways that we can keep meeting our core patient education goals. To continuously cultivate and maintain our commitment to the FootEducation Mission, this website's content is peer-reviewed by our stellar editors, each of whom is a well-respected orthopedic foot and ankle surgeon.

The type of information you will find on FootEducation includes:

Easy to understand information on a comprehensive list of foot and ankle conditions

Descriptions of all common foot and ankle surgeries
A powerful tool for identifying which conditions cause pain in various areas of the foot

A review of basic information that will help patients better understand diagnosis and treatment of foot and ankle problems.

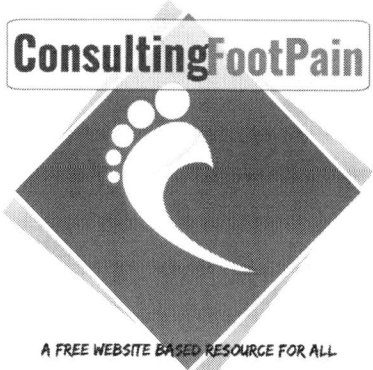

Shutterstock/talitha_it

Consulting foot pain (CFP) is a brand name and uses similar formats to other sites but UK podiatrists can contribute material. Both sites are impartial, sell nothing and have free access. The CFP site uses the FE site for surgical advice as well as NHS, NICE and other specialist sites from the UK and USA.

Articles

Articles and information need to be informative but not burdened with heavy jargon. Ideally they should offer a range of options. Sites such as FootEducation.com, BoFAS and some material within the College of Podiatry sites are biased toward surgery. The PASCOM site previously mentioned publishes annual reports using large datasets. Data requires careful interpretation before being shared with patients. CFP uses case histories and anecdotes to add dimension to the subject. It makes sense to use free linked sites and put them on your own website selecting material of value and using the http:// links. However, if you don't have time, you could engage someone to write for your practice. This may be new for many and is innovative without threat and can accelerate your brand. As material grows more can be shared with everyone. See chapter 11 for further ideas where I discuss Reedsy.com as an example. It is important to invest money where it allows you to optimise your clinical expertise.

BRAND SELF-HELP

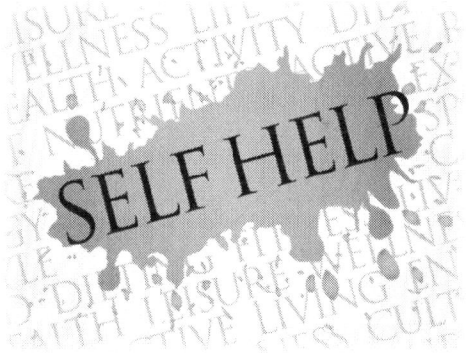

Shutterstock/dizain

We live in a world where there is so much for free, especially with published literature, that we have to compete on a similar basis. The difference that podiatrists can make for patients is by offering *self-*

help advice. Streamlining foot care in this way assures you they have done everything possible.

Sometime ago I saw the idea that writing a book for GPs would provide a helpful guide for their patients. I did this locally after giving a talk to several GP groups.

Podiatry is not a profession that self generates literature in abundance except from the professional bodies and around the Foot Health promotion dates. It has only been a recent change that videos and social media have increased to promote the image. To date no current study is available to show the impact of this social *mediarizing* effect in our field.

The profession has the ability to do more, but it needs authors and confident promotors. British podiatrists strengths lie with research but this only has a small contributing group set around university and NHS educational posts. Translating research even to general podiatrists is something that the profession as a whole must recognise as important. On the ground general podiatrists need to promote research and findings to promote the benefit of podiatric care and to show why patients should go to podiatrists as first line foot carers.

Hard Sell

In the USA there is no shortage of budding authors. A cornucopia of material exists although a good deal focuses on hard sell.

This happens by way of reading information which provides tantalising promises. The reader perseveres and reaches the end only to find that the material of any value now costs money or the tag attached. Because English is the primary language of the internet it is easy to be drawn in by false promises and pseudo-advertising.

Many authors that write about feet are not even podiatrists but exercise gurus, psychoanalysts and some with spurious professional pedigrees. When analysed the advice is basic, unscientific and cannot hope to consider the complexities of pathology or patient need.

Influential publications

One of the first books I bought and read for self help was the Running Foot Doctor published in paperback by a DPM. It was a good read and really elevated the podiatrist's role in that sphere back in 1981. In 1976 however, my first borrowed book from the then London Foot Library was a book to do with looking after feet. This was the portal into the world of unknown podiatry at a time when the only term that existed was 'chiropody'.

In Australia there has been an upsurge in branded books on business practice. In the UK we are not exploiting any dominance in this market. Quality books on studies in elements of practice yes, but these are academic heavies and will appeal to the educational career markets more than clinicians of podiatry or their patients. They are written for students and housed in libraries often with a high price tag.

> When Churchill-Livingstone (now Elsevier) took over my own two text books, written for undergraduate students, the price tag was high at £38 at the time (1995-97) for a hard cover and inevitably was passed down to the next generation with a reduced price tag. Of course this in itself was entrepreneurial. Later editions were cosmetic and so this actually did not matter to the whiley student who was happy to bypass the newer edition as doubtless the difference was perceived as marginal between a new and old copy. This system actually diminished sales of the later editions and is a salutary lesson to authors where larger groups of readers can effect change.

This short anecdote highlights book price tags for the average person's pocket. E-books have done much to lower the price and can be offered in colour and have the advantage of hyperlinking to other useful sites. However, not everyone is geared to information technology. Those with low information technological skills will need paper and be able to download files.

Soft sell

Did you know that one of the best ways of promoting your product is to find the soft sell? Tell a story. Appeal to someone in a different way. This means not directly but present a product that tells a story with a good ending.

> A woman damaged her toe at work. As she worked for the local bank, and they cared they found my general practice. Health and safety had not reached the heights it has today and back then, 1983, the chance of litigation was small. The bank paid for her treatment invoiced at £25.00[18]. She had ripped her nail on the edge of a filing cabinet. I anaesthetised the toe to make it comfortable, resected the torn nail and dressed this. The time period associated with damage to treatment was an hour. I had in fact acted as an A&E (minor trauma unit). All was well and the lady returned to see me for a follow up delighted at the swift response. The soft sell is not that we can do this, or can do that, but this is what can be done by example.

The story needs to be real and relates to humanity. Some humour helps as you are raising the boundaries of communication to fit in with the context of real life.

---

[18] This was the price charged in 1982 and included a local anaesthetic and minor procedure when a new consultation = £6.50 in an old lace town in the North Midlands area where the average consultation was between £3.50 – £5.00

The Blogger

The blog is a great mechanism to achieve story telling and here I am referring to the anecdote. Many podiatrists use social media. The downside is that patients and public can comment adversely and if you fail to scrutinise this regularly such a message may do harm. Here is an anecdote providing an example.

> My wife hated history at school because it was about rote learning. *Dates and facts that seemed to have no relevance.* She loves social history where she can apply history to real life. When Richard III was found to have become part of a car park this raised her level of interest beyond the so called hunch back king, even if the caricature was probably created by Shakespeare.

Web content

If you set up a website, what are you trying to do with it? Provide location or times of opening? What you do or offer, who you are and who you work with. For most this is cheap and cost effective and requires little maintenance. Gregory says that

> your website is the most important marketing tool you have for business growth and brand building. This is the place that your consumers will visit to learn more about your business, and take action when they are ready.
>
> Not only does the user experience have to be exceptional in order to convert, but your

messaging needs to tell your brand story. It's
important to have all the right pieces in place
when first launching your website.

If you do use a website, you need to become
familiar with search engine optimisation (SEO)
which is a learned skill and takes a while to focus
on. SEO helps drive content toward higher viewer
ranking. The six websites that I selected in the next
chapter were all driven with the SEO in mind and
picked out by searching. This is exactly what a
patient will do when trying to find someone. SEO is
based on headings, explanations and the way in
which content is written. I use *WordPress*, one of
many such web platforms and this provides a traffic
light system for the strength of your blog or article.

The advice given is to start with a strong heading,
add focus keywords as well as tags. A focus key
word would typically be a word most used in both
the heading and article. The tag would be a category
of the article such as *feet*, or *pain* or *podiatry.* Too
many words, long sentences, insufficient
hyperlinking, too few headings to break up
paragraphs will all affect the strength that
WordPress considers appropriate for the SEO. The
SEO comes into its own once the first few searches
are made and become a repeatable heading. This is
by far preferred than paying to boost your SEO.

Reflection by Survey

Having written for podiatrists under 'reflective
practice', it was time to analyse my work over the

last two years. Reflecting upon what you do in regard to promotion is important as you want to make sure you are targeting the right people. Using surveys to do this is not easy because we are inundated with feedback in modern society. If you receive 25% returns, then you are doing well. Any type of feedback allows you to make adjustments and if you act upon the feedback then you are truly reflecting.

By Post

Postal surveys are almost dead and ineffective unless you are prepared to invest money, provide return as pre-paid postage on addressed envelopes. An incentive works but skews the response immediately. The internet provides many methods to acquire data but you need e-mail addresses and that opens up the whole can of worms under GDPR or general data protection regulation. There are many books on surveys and it best to use short statements and focus on what you need.

Patient Satisfaction

My best survey called PSQ-10 was developed in 1992, only it had no name at the time. The purpose behind the survey was to follow up patient treatment as part of an audit system. This became known as Podiatric Audit in Surgical Outcome

Measurement, better known as **PASCOM-10**. The 'ten' was added when the database went on-line in 2010 as a web-based system. The use of scaled answers (0-10) is easy to respond to but has no rationale. As a quick and ready method it provides an idea of attitude because people tend to react instantly and this reflects their immediate thought without thinking. The open box response is less popular because people have to think, and even write!

The bulleted responses for options works for narrow fields, but irritates the user who feels that not all options are available. PSQ-10 was tested in house, then nationally amongst podiatrists and then was reviewed by two colleagues independently (Taylor et al 2008). Additionally, it was then used in an Egyptian study by an orthopaedic author. Patient satisfaction questionnaire ten had more value than traditional audit tools, i.e before and after measurement because it was available and accessible to the user. The results of the questionnaire can be used by professionals to show their results. This comes back to the soft sell. Show don't tell. Evidence speaks volumes.

Paid advertising

Paying to advertise is hit and miss although using standard advertising still is probably worthwhile. Yellow Pages is of course on-line and easy to access. Don't forget patients who leave a bad review can have a negative effect on future clients.

If you have enough business don't advertise. If your referral source is strong enough, don't advertise. Save money for making that brand work. If you are starting up, then advertising is a necessary requirement, but an article that can be published might be better. Find that new angle. Chapter 11 provides a few more tips on the subject of advertising using a website.

Get out and give talks

Get out and give talks 'Projecting Your Image' is my new contribution to all would be public speakers, so help is not far away. I have talked at meetings with groups such as the Round Table (albeit around a square table), GPs surgeries, at restaurants, hotels, conference centres, Women's Institute meetings held in village halls. Short and well produced talks allow room for plenty of questions. In fact, if you can engineer a talk so that 50% of the length is given to question time you can market your brand very effectively. I would always find new patient referrals increased after a talk.

FOOT HEALTH PROMOTION

As a calendar event Foot Health has been promoted by the College of Podiatry and encourages many practises to get out and be seen actively. The first *Foot Health Week* was held in 1983. As a branch officer of the then Society of Chiropodists[19] we found funds to produce enlarged colour photos, which went into shop windows. Without personal computers this was challenging and colour production expensive. I went onto BBC Radio Stoke and gave an interview. I drew on my passion for podiatry but looking back I needed a wealth of case history anecdotes and experience as I was still very young and new to the ways of publicity. In truth we all were naïve as one of our committee a future successful Chair of Council would recall only too well some 25 years later. The early days of 'biomechanics' was just emerging but a far cry from the arena of MSK today.

With social media, videos, podcasts, the opportunity for promotion is readily available. *Podiatry Now* and *Podiatry Review* report progress but then look at 2020 and how an event such as Covid-19 can ambush efforts. It is difficult to talk about feet and foot health when a nation sees escalating mortality figures and its Prime Minister brought down, and yet people have started walking more than ever!

Budgets & Give-Aways

If you do pay for any advertising campaign always set a budget and review the benefit before repeating the exercise. Change direction if necessary and

---

[19] The Society of Chiropodists changed its name after incorporation with the Podiatry Association and Association of Chief Chiropody Officers in 1997

accept the learning curve. Returning to the idea of articles. These are often called blogs, the videos called vlogs. Giving something away is often a powerful call as mentioned earlier. Free consultations can work but don't use these if you have plenty of business. Advice through a website is easier to control, but set limitations. Ideally give away a bit and drive people to your market place.

Printed material can work well providing referral information for patients with practice details. Leaflets with your practice name, e-mail address, website and telephone number are fine if you have a disposable budget. Headed paper and cards are still a valid tool to help promote your brand and are very inexpensive today with modern on-line printing. But, shop around for printing sources.

Your message must be understood. Brands need to be visible. You ideally want to be the GO TO PERSON for that foot problem.

Important material should include:

> Who you are. Qualifications, profile, personal attributes, an anecdote about your ability can all help. The balance between bragging (hubris) and positive promotion can be difficult.

COMMUNICATION ETIQUETTE

The personal computer has made life easier to write letters. In fact, today, dictation can be achieved without secretaries, although if you have a busy practice, a receptionist, telephone operator and secretary are worth their weight in terms of effective communication of your brand. The front face of your organisation is best served by a kind voice and one that seeks to help and support enquiry. A good receptionist can affect a practice exponentially. As my work became more complex I relied on my secretaries who I placed an enormous value on to promote my brand, and answer every query politely and efficiently.

Here are two anecdotes that reflect on broken etiquette.

Referral

The first golden rule in referring to anyone is to write a letter couched in the correct style on headed paper, typed, dated and signed.

> A colleague would often send me patients. First the telephone would ring imploring me to undertake a surgical procedure as this was not her field. Likewise, I would refer her cases requiring orthoses by typed letter.
>
> The patient would turn up with a crumpled note with her practice heading and compliment slip.
>
> The note was usually hand written in small writing but was all too brief and seldom lacked substance.
>
> 'I would be so grateful if you would see this sweet lady for me she has an awful IGTN I cannot do anything more for her.'

This would be one of the better notes!

> On one occasion I needed evidence that a bone
> fide referral had been made and no record could
> be found (4 years after the event). This ended up
> costing me no less than £800.00 to defend
> myself!

This is a salutary lesson and I changed my policy in requiring a typed referral setting out the correct information and headed with - name, DoB, main complaint and most importantly what had been done by the podiatrist up to that data. My secretary would be asked to chase this up, but it led to some inconvenience for patients and made me look bad rather than my colleague.

Letters are as much part of the official records and the clinical notes. Without this platform page legal defense is weakened.

Response

It is an absolute golden rule to write to anyone referring you a patient to thank them. It is useful to share a second anecdote.

This story is **HOW NOT TO;**

> A colleague was referred a patient by a consultant
> (orthopaedic surgeon). The letter sent back by the
> colleague, while intending to be helpful, was
> badly framed. It pointed out the consultant's
> treatment had to be addressed as by inference it
> was sub-optimal. A list of the faults with his
> management were thus described. The consultant

O.S came to me to ask if this was an acceptable standard, quite apart from being very upset.

Every time someone reads your professional report based on your correspondence, your advice will be recognised as a point of authority. Your brand will grow from here. I can say that the story above damaged this podiatrist's practice and was an example of the worst hubris and poor etiquette observed in my many years of practice. Not least my colleague was a senior consultant.

It is mandatory within the framework of good etiquette to let anyone with a common (clinical) interest in your patient's foot problem know that they are seeing you. This avoids any conflict later on. It goes without saying that the patient GP must always be informed.

Clients and Competitors

Of course you have competition. Your first competitor is also your main client, the GP. But he or she is also your largest competitor as he is also contracted as a self-employed professional with the NHS scheme.

How does he become a competitor and client?
Your GP is provided with an annual fee for his case load based around the number of patients on the books. If a patient is seen often, the unit remuneration goes down. If a patient is rarely seen, financially this is a bonus. If the GP undertakes certain promotional screenings, or undertakes

specific approved treatment, then additional payment is provided. So if a practice offers the same treatment as you and is paid to invest back into the practice for a given treatment plan, then you won't get the business as it makes no financial sense. If the practice however refers a patient to an NHS outlet for the same treatment that you can do, you may see that business, or not, depending upon your bid for commissioning treatment. As with any business the GP wants his money to go further.

To beat the system, you have to be better organised. You need to show you can provide a cost effective service. A robust audit and trail of satisfied patients can make a difference. Many patients will pay for treatment if they lose faith elsewhere, unless their finances are dire. When it comes to selecting a podiatrist, the GP will use some of the above, but also select the ones that he knows are reliable.

Always be helpful but be prepared to pass a patient onto someone else early if you cannot provide that service: -

'Look, I can't help you anymore but this man can.'

The referral comes to you because of knowledge of reliability from past experience. Although conscious of false praise, when a patient turned up and said, that *I came highly recommended* it was a pleasant start to the consultation. A letter that said *'please see and do your magic,'* equally told the story of confidence, even if I had no magic to offer! So in our business, brands do not always have to be visible but they are recognised by others.

The Importance of Access

It is important to be accessible. We once used pagers and answer phones. These still have a place but on-line booking makes more sense. Now we have text and e-mail facilities. When I looked at those random websites earlier I was pleasantly surprised to see some using an on-line booking system. This option gives patients control and is part of that all important presentation. A new patient who cannot contact you will go elsewhere but even if you are unable to help it is good to have made a good contact which will be remembered positively. Decide if you want to offer an out of hours service. This might mean adjusting your week; early or late. Don't do both on the same day.

Share

Share your on-call out of hours service especially where you provide skin and nail surgery. You don't want someone turning up at A&E unnecessarily. This is tougher when starting out. If your practice is multi-chair, then you can afford to spread the workload. But the message is share where you can to promote podiatry so you all benefit.

Be accessible by mobile, or at the end of a phone or text message. This is becoming part of successful practice but it does come with a cost to personal freedom and a balance has to be met.

Closing Thoughts About Information

In closing it is worthwhile making the point that as much of your care delivery is also about advice. The information that you use should be current and gained from as many reliable sites in addition to your clinical knowledge. Your experience drives your product. External information validates your advice.

In no particular order find the best site for the information you need? Decide how it is delivered and if you can pass it on unadulterated to your patient. Unlike scientific papers, fact sheets and smaller articles on key conditions can be of immense value as take away information for patients to digest.

All the sites mentioned have their own value and their links can be imported into your website or copied for patients to use. The *NHS* site within Trusts form the best all round sites for patient generic information, often with podiatry units publishing excellent material.

'Footeducation' as a site is valuable for quality impartial information but biased toward surgery.

The College of Podiatry (CoP) can vary enormously but worth reviewing under the patient's site rather than members. Remember only members can access this site and it is easy to think this reflects what the outside world can see. Likewise, the Institute of Chiropody & Podiatry (IOCP) varies in detail and has a smaller patient information resource.

OSGO, CoP and IOCP will support the podiatrist in terms of information to disseminate commercial but professionally designed literature. BoFAS presents professional viewpoints on a range of conditions but is limited to surgery in general and adopts generic views about foot conditions.

CFP is a new concept website for podiatry and still developing. Information varies between routine and surgical conditions with a bias toward self-help and routine. Pathology still requires specialist diagnosis and some lesser known treatment pathways and like all information sites there is still a limit as to how far written or verbal advice can be given without direct face to face.

9: Logos, Branding, Strap line

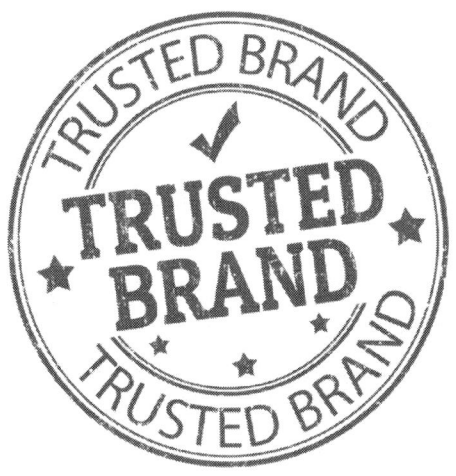

Shutterstock/ducu59us

Of the now 14,000 podiatrists there will be many who have bought into a business model framework optimising good management principles. Practice management is about efficiency and effectiveness, delivering what works, what supports the running of the practice and meeting all the standard requirements associated with safety and professional delivery. Independent practice subsumes majority of podiatrists with those in NHS England falling by 12%, reported in the House of Commons (2010). So this fall is hardly new. Single handed practice can be successful but those who have embraced multi-practice locations and staff employment can reach bigger audiences. In these circumstances branding is even more important. I was impressed in 2018 at the National CoP conference where I could see many podiatrists were already geared up with good attitudes toward business. They had probably taken courses to expand their skill set in business, others had a natural incline toward business acumen.

While professional bodies have a financial budget for advertising, this can only be used for generic promotion for its membership. Efforts at converting research to podiatry promotion are difficult, not least because they often don't optimise all podiatry and may focus on limited areas of our work. Inevitably those that are perceptive will need to do something to meet their own objectives. On the flip side many practitioners are happy to use generic promotion. Staying within one's comfort zone can cause stagnation and it is important to step outside this mystical boundary.

However, where academic papers exist and demonstrate a need for foot health content these should be edited for promotion to a lay readership (primordial cascading). Once research identifies a positive benefit or need, the brand can be attached to the facts and developed into publicity. So let's delve into websites further. An independent practice does not develop on its own. Some multi practices can now hit turnovers of six figures according to College of Podiatry. Podiatry is a good profession to be in and has a capable earning power. But it needs hard work and perspicacity. I looked at a random group of websites to find out if strap lines or brand messages were being used as part of podiatry. All were *accessed on 4 November 2019* for my series on branding for reflective podiatric practice.

A Quick Google

I hit my search engine for websites on podiatry and selected the first six that I came across.

Here are the results

One used a strap line
Two had defined logos
All six had clear and colourful landing pages.
All stated their range of treatment.
One site used a selection of headers that changed after a short period in sequence. This covered 4 areas; hypermobility, orthopaedics, paediatrics and sports.

Of the six:

three focused on the title podiatry alone

the other <u>three</u> emphasised their business as chiropody.

In the box over the page I have listed some thoughts focusing on these landing pages. All had clean lines, i.e not unduly cluttered. They were comprehensive but gave a different perspective of the profession. Locations varied; South West, North East, London, Home Counties, East Midlands and East Anglia. While this was not a scientific survey, selection was random. Each had a strong *Search Engine Optimization* (SEO). Of the six websites one emphasised diabetes. The full range of practice treatment available was shown. Some sites focused on a key area such as the one emphasising 'musculoskeletal podiatrists'.

The only strap line found stated;

OPEN THE RIGHT DOOR TO HEALTHY FEET.

Most podiatrists brand small areas of podiatric practice rather than clear subject headings, although diabetes was clearly sign posted as was 'MSK'. From the content of the websites four observations can be made. Think *public* not podiatry. Try to engage the public in new concepts about feet so as to provide some education within your advert and web page. A patient requires a podiatrist to help them sift through a number of possible conditions that even the GP may not be familiar with. Ideally no problem should last more than a few days.

149

There is a tendency to mix up terms. Bespoke and prescription are both made to measure. It would be better to say made to measure, or custom made.

Paediatric or childhood problems. While the first reference might sound better, the second is less confusing than paediatric medicine and so childhood is clearer. Podiatric and paediatric are often confused.

Arch and ball pain. Of all these listed areas this one is perhaps the most direct but might be worthy of clearer sign-posting as arch and ball are well known locations for different pain problems in the foot. The reason to consult a podiatrist is to exclude other problems so you might want to show why diagnosis is difficult and different treatment might be required for each condition.

Arch pain may relate to fasciitis, poor tendon function or degenerative changes.
Ball pain might be associated with nerve entrapment, skin complaints such as corns, arthritis, bone fractures and toe deformity

We then come to locations as forefoot, midfoot and rearfoot pain. Why not foot and ankle pain? The foot is chiefly divided into the ball (as above) and middle of the foot consisting of the arch. The ankle works with the heel bone.

Website Promotion of Podiatry

Corns and calluses
Ingrowing toe nail
Fungal nail
Gait related problems
Full biomechanical assessment
Bespoke, prescription orthoses (1)
Diabetic foot assessments
Nail braces
Cosmetic podiatry
Paediatric podiatry / childhood conditions
(2)
Hydrotherapy
Sports injury
Peripheral arterial disease
Rheumatoid arthritis
Abnormal nails
Heel pain
Arch and ball pain (3)
Bunions and other toe deformities
Forefoot, midfoot and rearfoot conditions4
Hip & spine

Taken from a short random survey using Google search
engine. November 2019
(1 to 3 are discussed in the box on the previous page.)

Combining strap lines with logos

CARING FOR FOOT HEALTH

In my practice I used the tag/strap line above.

Visual imaging comes to mind first *when* you think of a brand. When I came to consider a logo for Busypencilcase Communications I certainly did not have the expertise or artistic flare to design my own. I set a budget and found some people who specialised. The net result was a name tag and logo with a healthcare image. My strap or tag line became

PROGRESS THROUGH THE ART OF COMMUNICATION

My focus was communication. Without communication in professional practice we cannot make progress and so communication represents a skill that needs to be developed. 'Skill' however would have been too long, despite only four letters but 'ART', at three letters made a good substitute because speaking and writing words is a craft as much as a science. You can make your own logo if you have the time and skill, but a well designed logo will last a lifetime if you achieve what you want and need.

Colours and background are all important to make your logo unique. The websites I selected in the snapshot study for this article all had good colour combinations. Using people in photo shots is far better than names alone. Do make sure that photos are cropped and professionally taken. This is where paying out is worthwhile. The message you want to convey is;

> LOOK, I'M FRIENDLY, RELAXED AND I WELCOME YOU. YOU ARE IN SAFE HANDS

Why have a logo?

A sign that is clear and recognisable like the Amazon A-Z / smiley face means you translate the image faster without reading each word. **Eric Bergman** a Canadian media training consultant, uses an analogy, Bergman's Miles.

If when driving from Birmingham to London one would not pass a sign that says;

> IF YOU MAINTAIN AN AVERAGE SPEED OF SEVENTY MILES PER HOUR, YOU SHOULD REACH LONDON IN APPROXIMATELY 2.571 HOURS.

The sign would actually say -

**London
180
miles**

This illustrates the point about minimal word use. Signs indicating distances use numbers rather than words. The same information is used but in a different way. Knowing the distance, you can calculate the time based on your average speed. Add an image that conveys information and the processing is faster. In the case of the car, one would just use the satnav!

Consider the instant recognition of a label like the MacDonalds brand. If you travelled to St Petersburg you can identify with a known standard of reliability, in other words, you know what to expect. I am not suggesting or recommending MacDonald's here, only using this as an example of successful branding. In the same way the NHS conveys reliability, free at the point of access, no fuss and pleasant people. But contrast this with expectations in the independent sector.

Perceptions of the Independent Sector

- You go to the independent sector because you have medical insurance cover. Why not; you pay in monthly.
- You avoid the NHS if you want treatment on your terms, at a time of your choosing and don't want to wait long.
- You want to sit down in a pleasant waiting room and know that you will be treated as a precious client not a number.
- You like the free coffee and biscuits; that personal touch. The place smells clean.
- All the staff look neat and uniforms are less confusing than the NHS.
- A small area for tiny tots complete with toys and coloured books is available.

This perception is maintained by some but not all independent hospitals. The NHS often matches some of these elements, but its budget is designed toward front line care, not frippery. In the NHS the quality of care is the part that the public accept, not least as there are few hidden costs. The NHS as a brand is and has been powerful but struggles with conflicting image and delivery. Prime Minister Blair tried to brand the NHS with individuality between Trusts. The individual identity from Trust to Trust cost enormous sums that were reversed later on. Political meddling is expensive when not thought through, even if the intentions are well meaning. The next example however was a master plan in advertising, mixing essential advice with balanced propaganda, a clear message and call to action[20]. During the Corona virus pandemic, the NHS became the front line 'war effort' and was optimally branded by Downing Street and endorsed by science. The logo has always been three letters in block italics NHS.

The genesis of the message can be traced to a Zoom conference call by Lee Cain, Boris Johnson's director of communications, on the afternoon of Thursday March 19, just as the government was moving towards imposing lockdown. Hope & Dixon (2020)

The words below were crafted onto a yellow background with a dashed red edged band appearing like radioactive tape. This became the logo embroidered by the words -

The strap line was powerful together with the narrative made from seven words in three distinct sentences used on every media device that existed.

Where Do You Use Logos?

Logos go on office fronts, business cards, headed paper, your information sheets, maybe your clinical clothing. They identify your brand, provide instant recognition, professionalism, knowledge that the

---

[20] History doubtless will judge these events as much still unfolds at the time of writing when this author was in Lockdown himself!

logo stands for a service that is reliable, effective, price sensitive, assured, regulated and believes in you as a number 1 priority. Well, the last paragraph is your aim. Stick a fantastic logo on your door and it won't mean anything if you don't work at it. So how do you work at it?

You need to deliver a message, but to who? Target your audience.

Gregory (2019) suggests that the foundation for a brand is based on your target audience meaning, who exactly you are trying to reach?

Is it people in pain, those who suffer from walking disability, those who cannot find footwear to fit a grossly deformed foot? Finding the specific key also includes the 'buyer audience'. You might think of this as those who buy into the product. For many seeing footcare as a 'product' belittles the professional view, and yet to ignore the fact we are all salespeople is to take a naïve attitude. Head in the sand approach! Look at the following audience profiles.

- Age
- Gender
- Location
- Income
- Education Level

The mission might be to meet the needs of all of these groups in general practice, but if one specialises the groups inevitably shrink. The strange psychology is that once you have a target audience life is easier as you find you can really dig deep and learn so much more. However, you will need people to test your product and build some testimonials.

Printed Materials

Printing is still expensive even in this day and age of digital print. Save printing for those areas that you feel you need to promote. A classic example is keeping personal leaflets designed where you cannot acquire leaflets elsewhere. See each of your main treatment themes as a product for promotion.

Give patients a chance to consider the treatment options and support this with a colour leaflet; outcome = information.

HOW TO GO ABOUT TESTIMONIALS

A testimonial can be included together with your name, your brand, a strap or tag line, contacts and so forth. A patient leaving with information is powerful and can be passed on. In the aforementioned survey I found no testimonial but I did locate one from a Foot Health Practitioner[21]. We all know that testimonials are easy to fudge and as such some are provided by close friends and even colleagues. Living in a world where we are all cautious about our personal details being exposed, there are methods to protect from this risk. I use the

---

[21] A Foot Health Practitioner (FHP) delivers foot health care at a different level to registered podiatrists but there is overlap.

following example. Ben is the podiatrist (*name made up*).

> Ben Solomon treated a condition I never
> thought I would get rid of. He has given me
> my life back. *Greta Finchley*. Contact 0121-
> 459-1234 / e-mail Sole.podcare@gmail.com

The testimonial is powerful because it is emotional and can be used with patient permission. Use Greta's real name but if not, ask what she might like to be called. This is the fun bit. Greta could use a name she wished her parents had given her, so her name still remains anonymous. Next you need to validate the testimonial. That is to ensure it was not made up. Maybe 10% of patients might be willing to give their real contact telephone or e-mail, but don't count on it. Use your own contact details so that you can screen people if Greta has agreed to allow you to pass her information on. Here is another tip that I found. Find a testimonial that is negative.

> Ben Solomon worked hard to help my foot.
> Sadly, I was not cured and I had to see a
> specialist, but I was grateful to him for doing his
> best and finding someone who could help. He
> advised me that he always tried to prevent
> surgery for becoming necessary but sometimes it
> doesn't work that way.

This is brimming with positive vibes for a testimonial. Why? Ben publishes it. He is honest and recognises that he is not perfect. The reader can see that integrity is part of the practice. Lastly he influenced the outcome positively.

Negative can be made positive!

When I posted a negative response, similar to the one above, feedback was encouraging. This type of honesty equates to integrity and probity. You will need evidence that you see a good number of people i.e evidence from counting.

Once back at home if you shut the door and forget about your practice you will commit a folly against yourself. This is the 21st century and you cannot afford to allow competitors a jump. There is always something to do. Review, prepare, plan and execute is a simple enough mantra but if you don't look at targets, numbers, effectiveness, income over expenditure the business side will fail. Time has to be allocated outside the workface of podiatry. You will need to show what your market offers (type of treatment). Data has always provided the power to evaluate activity and the action of performing this task is called audit. Use a reliable database to collect essential statistics.

Making Decisions

- What area of specialty are you best at?
- Which group of patients / clients do you see most?

The balance between being successful and generating income are never far apart. Consider removing something that has a high cost with low benefit to your practice. In my own practice I removed treating children and orthotic work. I was best at diagnostic problem solving, injection treatment and surgery. As time passed, the surgical procedures that were less effective and cost disproportionately and had more risks for recovery were squeezed out.

Referral

While the example above applied to me as a podiatric surgeon, I could equally have altered my business if I had not been undertaking surgery. For everything you give up you find a new niche. The importance is not to lose business but to stratify your expertise. Decisions are based on the reality of activity and so your data needs to be accurate. I would point out that I loved dealing with children, but the hospital I worked for made it almost impossible for this to work or have value. Such decisions may take time, but you have to be pragmatic in business.

When you do not provide a service but use someone else chose a reliable source as this is still part of your active participation.

> I once referred a child to an orthopaedic surgeon
> because they were in pain and at the time my
> service could not offer the corrective surgery
> required. Two years later the mother and her

child, now in her mid teens, returned to see me and their unhappiness was palpable. I felt enormous remorse at not searching wider but I had used an orthopaedic website to make my decision.

Reflection came in the shape of expanding our scope and service to manage the flat foot surgically without the need to refer out.

BLOGGING

Blogs are great. Short articles on foot conditions can enhance websites and connect to those who are interested in your product. I started blogging on my website in 2014 and found it really helpful to tie in factsheets, self-help sheets as well as articles that related to anonymised patients. These eventually gave way to my first book, but then this is not something you need to concern yourself with, although the power of a small information booklet is worth producing. The booklet is a conduit to GP practices and other referrers as well as give-aways for your patients. I would not recommend selling published materials unless that is a clear direction you want to go in. Most UK produced materials come under those academics who do this for a living. Working with Busypencilcase Communications Ltd I can tell you that the process of writing and publishing is not for the feint hearted.

Blogs have to be updated but the fun thing is that you can link them as your content builds. Video blogging or *vlogging* is now the rage as it is portable and provides bite size chunks. Great for the youthful section of society but we still see a large proportion of people, age wise, who do not favour these more portable methods.

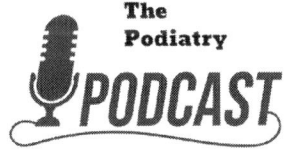

The other medium worth exploring as mentioned earlier is the Podcast, a recording of your voice providing information. This makes information very much more personal if the patient knows you. I come back to the view that 'we' as a body think the professional body should promote us? Yes, of course they should, after all we pay their salaries. And yet what can they do without our expertise? Taking charge of our own brand must become an important part of our work.

10: Giving Credit to our Brand

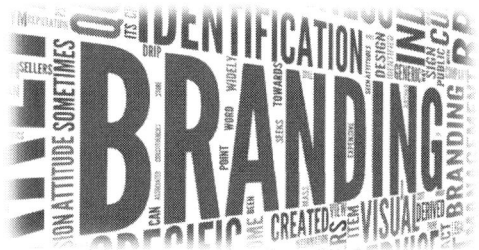

Shutterstock/Rafal Olechhowksi

LET'S GET CRITICAL

Branding is reflected within your advertising strategy but it is larger than advertising alone. Branding is much about yourself but also how others perceive your ability. You cannot rely on your professional body to do the work for you. It is important to contribute in such a way as to influence and support professional bodies to work on your behalf. It is all too easy to place responsibility at someone else's doorstep. Tony Gavin makes Brand even clearer in his own mind. He says,

'Brand is just reputation, that is all it is, but the word brand gets quite mixed up in the idea of commercial propositions. I think the reputation of podiatry is the absolute responsibility of everyone and every single podiatrist and provided (that) they are doing something with the utmost integrity and effort to be the very best that it can be in the space they are working and choose to do, then podiatry has a very very bright future. The problem for our brand and reputation comes when we don't own it as collective individuals. When we externalise reputation as a problem of the brand of podiatry and think it is (as just) something out there. None of us would look to other people to improve because we understand that accountability lies completely with us as an individual and I think that's how we (must) solve any problem within podiatry.'

Quantifiable components such as educational credits, qualifications and experience are pillars associated with primary branding; but there is a soft power that needs to be harnessed. Telling someone that you have a first class honours degree won't be of much help in private practice and less so without experience. Showing evidence of performance provides greater credibility. Brand is associated with image, based on visual and verbal identity, reputation and what people think of you. One big question is what should podiatry stand for? I wanted to be good at everything and treat anything footy! This is neither brandable but steeped in naiveté, despite the good intentions of a podiatrist qualified with a narrow spectrum of practice in 1978. When making GCSE decisions at 13, students need to know what career to follow. Decisions at this age are not easy or come instantly.

An apprenticeship, once considered important for all careers, is slowly re-emerging although the idea never went away entirely. The idea that you can go to university and expect your qualification to provide instant access to a sustainable living has been a big disappointment to many graduates in other fields. This is because it is easy to misunderstand what university stood for. It is a vehicle for building on life. If you have a vocational qualification such as podiatry you can turn this into an instant career generating a decent income. However, just having a vocational career is not the end, it is still the beginning. Like trainee medics who pass through specialist programmes, it is important to sample the whole range of sub-specialties. There are several reasons why this is important.

Firstly, we all need to know what the whole spectrum looks like as we need to recognise different skill sets that can be built upon after we qualify.

Secondly, and of equal importance, the decision to select which sub-specialty you are most attracted to can have an impact later on. As with GCSE selection some do not make the right decision but this is part of life's big tapestry of choice, trial and error. It is important to not be too disappointed as knowledge can always be applied in ways we often are unaware of at the time of initial participation.

Even in general (podiatry) practice this becomes important. It can be helpful to develop a sub-specialty to make yourself more marketable. Eventually this might become your potential brand for your future but only when you find your niche. The box below shows the principle areas of podiatry that are brandable although 'general' comes with caveats. That is limitations of scope and a requirement to use a referral model. The referral model relates to a recognition that you have a responsibility to prepare your patient for another stage in their management process.

Branding Podiatry

Sports (MSK)
Medical (at risk)
Surgical (focused on podiatric surgery)
Children (podo-paediatrics)
General (general population support for foot health)
Elderly (home support and clinic, mobility and tissue preservation)

NHS Opportunities

The career structure after qualifying is still relatively new. Much of the evidence for this is outside the remit of this book. However, the extended scoping of podiatry has been an important lever to change the NHS career ladder.

Wastage of education leads to resentment, but lost skills and acquisitions whilst training toward podiatric surgery should become brandable within the NHS. To be clear this can only work where specific education goals have been met. A working example is best exemplified by the process through Podiatric training for foot surgery. It is possible to utilise part of the skills that would have acquired during the formative years between MSc and the initial surgical examinations. The Masters programme was created around 2003. Anyone who failed the extended surgery course would still gain a Masters qualification (MSc) provided that the degree course and dissertation had been completed. Within the NHS this would have gained credit, and it would be possible to attach this to a structured career divergence. Although perhaps of less application in the independent sector, where there is no career structure alongside this speciality, such arrangements within the NHS have lagged behind.

Discontinuing the fellowship has led to huge wastage and disappointment as well as resentment for some. In a few cases those podiatrists who failed to achieve their desires were able to convert to extended scope podiatrists and able to play a part in the MSK triage team. This has been an example of effective re-branding. When my own service was expediently shrunk, I moved to the independent sector and built a successful service supporting the very clients I had managed when within the NHS. However, a close colleague had to re-brand himself.

Possibly this could be regarded as an example of one the first established extended scope podiatrists in podiatric surgery. With twenty years' worth of skills experience he was adopted by the local orthopaedic team. This had been assisted because our podiatric surgery team had been adopted within the Orthopaedic Department over the previous 2 years. Not only was he welcomed but his skill set was of undeniable value to which he added an independent prescribing qualification. While this is a living and breathing example of good practice development, the professional body has not embraced the wider potential which undoubtedly would offer better collaboration with orthopaedics.

What We Do

If brand is you and your ability can be represented by the following mnemonic i.e seeking to maintain mobility as in M.A.I.D. Your unique selling proposition is easier to dovetail within this framework. MAID was discussed earlier where this set of objectives impact on mobility (M) by managing alignment (A), dealing with tissue integrity (I) and influencing pain or discomfort (D).

Shared practice

As with many GP practices, if these are built up with other colleagues you can spread your services across a greater area using people with different skill sets. You don't have to stick to one of the categories aforementioned but if you blend two or more, the potential is greater. Think of a promotional brand line that could represent you and colleagues. Given that podiatry competes amongst other health professionals, especially in the arena of orthotic management, trying to create an edge is important. While we can look at statistics from our websites and see which clients are 'hitting it', we need to be able to look at our case load and use this to our advantage.

What works best? What is reliable?

Not all treatment works for everyone. Never press someone for treatment. Provide them with options and use professionally produced leaflets and information give aways. Undoubtedly many will be available from your professional body. However, some are better being produced personally for your practice consumption. Kaputa (2013) suggests,

> We have all spent much time doing what we think others want us to do, rather than what we want to do.

The corollary is that we can support both our need and theirs by focusing on the ingredients of best practice. As a podiatrist with a surgical specialty I was fortunate. My brand was already created. I had an NHS base which is usually essential for all consultant practices.

It has been said, once a consultant retires from the NHS, his private practice fades quickly thereafter. I was fortunate that this did not happen to me as my brand was adopted by my private hospital and hence promoted amongst other services. My catchment, was large and around a population of one million throughout the region. My foot brand became ConsultingFootPain which competed well enough with my main competition; fellow podiatric and orthopaedic surgeons. But for most podiatrists this type of support has to be developed in a different way.

Podiatry does enjoy some independent hospital privileges and for the major hospital provider names in the UK, podiatrists often offer services in parallel with physiotherapy. This is a growing area of potential for single practitioners.

MANAGEMENT

Creating a positive perception of ourselves means that we cannot sit behind those age old laurels. The NHS back in the seventies and eighties offered wonderful opportunities. In some ironic way it was the inter play between competing Health Authorities, then Health Districts and later Health Trusts, that provided opportunities for staff to develop. Much came from an organisation called the Association of Chief Chiropody Officers (ACCO).

Disliked by some of the organisations, ACCO held a cohesiveness between NHS podiatry units until in 1997 the formation of the College saw the break up of both ACCO and the Podiatry Association. The resultant effect was brought together when, through the Camden Accord, the Society of Chiropodists started to embrace the title podiatry (SCP or SOCAP). The loss of ACCO, and hence competition may well have played a larger role in diluting the current position of podiatry in the NHS. Nonetheless other factors also come into play, not withstanding constant re-organisation and dropping grants from university education. The NHS podiatry workforce is at its lowest level since podiatrists started being employed following the state registration act 1960. The independent sector provides an easier route for self development not least as educational funds for staff development have shrunk with time. The benefit of independent practice has been that educational courses are tax deductible. Furthermore, each podiatrist can direct their own career. However, investment in time to develop scope has now fallen to the responsibility of individuals within the NHS. NHS employees will currently have to become proactive in seeking support grants due the the shrinkage of educational budgets

Working in group practices offers a better opportunity to build a strong collective. One of podiatry's weaknesses has always been not working within multi-disciplinary teams.

The acquisition of new skills is important to promote your brand and to fill any deficit in your service if it is within reach.

New clinical skills

Ultrasound diagnostics, therapeutic injections, extra-corporeal shock wave therapy, microwave treatment, and dermoscopy are relatively new options. Foot scanners are another development that practices can capitalise on as the unit cost has dropped. Gaining experience on the job and turning up to observe is now fraught with red tape and beaurocracy. What once was easy to expand clinical exposure after graduating has been impeded. Again this is a good reason to work in teams.

Competition for orthoses might be better challenged by reversing trends and using the approach of not providing prescription orthoses. Marketing inexpensive products and promoting the fact that over 90% of orthoses fit this market can be exploited. When you do reassess a patient for a Rx orthosis you are in an entirely stronger position if the initial work has not been disproportionately billed.

REFLECTING ON MEDICINE

It is good to have access to POM medicines, but podiatry was founded on the need to use skills that could minimise the use of oral medication. The net effect is that you can use the negative effect of overprescribing to your benefit. This is taking charge of your brand. Medicine to an extent and in contrast with podiatry has been too prescription orientated. In this first chapter I showed that poor time allocation and listening skills detracted from good care. The idea that patients leave with a script still has not been eradicated although cost containment of GP budgets has actually played a part in reducing the use of drugs.

Be different, don't copy

Podiatry needs to be different. It should not copy or imitate other services outside of the profession. Podiatry should focus on the fact it gives time to patients. To listen, to empathise and reflect. Contrast this to many GP practices today where they focus on 'numbers through'. You only have to read the previous Chair of the Royal College of General Practitioner's message about wasting time with computer interfaces to realise that one, Professor Helen Stokes-Lampard was fighting to put her profession back in the public's favour.

Medicine's Dilemma

Medicine is having a severe set back with a lack of new incomers. The loss of expertise from those born in the fifties and sixties who had worked the old system is impacting on the future of medical care at the face of health delivery. Incentives to retire early with generous pensions has been a recipe for a mass exodus to enjoy the fruits of labour, but problems sit deeper and gestate for the future. Reflect on medicines' fall from grace and look at your own profession of podiatry.

New ideas imported that scratch at the surface of the problem provides inadequate resolution. Inflexible protocols fail to address some of the more pressing matters in healthcare. The political basis upon which medicine has allowed itself to become driven has created change with irreparable harm. Once strong and a respected health care system, and envy of the world, only a misguided person might disagree with this analysis today. While pockets of innovation and superior service exist, these form a kaleidoscope of misleading images.

Make the Message Clear

Podiatry can at last enter the true medical field with new opportunities and if wise will use these to rebrand. Above all other professions, podiatry has a greater reach in educational, academic and clinical fields than many of the other allied health careers. Effective communication is important. I suggested that M.A.I.D utilises the four elements that best represent what podiatrists aim to achieve. Once you know your audience target then you can use the mnemonic to fit within a specific condition.

Reversing the mnemonic, one can promote *MAID* as **AID-M**. It is not necessary to explain MAID to all patients but within your communication you are using the evidence to achieve something that a patient will find beneficial and can relate to. Pain as discomfort (D), deformity and instability as alignment problems (A) and of course tissue problems as in integrity (I).

Take the management of pain for example in the case of IGTN. When using a phenolisation technique you might want to say that I can cure the problem, which might appear dubious at best because of the risk of failure. Promotion with integrity is essential in a profession based upon strong ethics. See the last sentence below.

> We have found that infection clears without an antibiotic. You can bathe the day after and care for the wound yourself without returning immediately. Should there be problems we are but a phone call away. The risks of reoccurrence are low but there is a possibility the problem might return.

OPPORTUNITY BRINGS CHANGE FOR DIFFERENT REASONS

There are many examples of successful promotion campaigns. The first example illustrates how to find the right message when you market a product. While this is unrelated to podiatry it serves as a useful case study.

> Pampers' developed a disposable nappy in the 1960s
> in the USA and was marketed as a time saving device
> for women. Cloth style nappies were seen as better
> for babies and so mothers voted to stay with the
> material best for their baby. The marketing failed.
> When Pampers altered their marketing message to
> that of better absorbency which benefitted babies this
> changed the purchasing perspective. Sales took off
> successfully. (Kaputa 2012)

Orthotics - Langer was a US based firm from New
York State, Long Island. Their factory unit was no
more impressive than any other unit that nestled in
this drab part of the islands' industrial complex, but
their product was. Langer came to the UK, saw a
market and realised there was potential. Sheldon
Langer and Justin Wernick provided UK podiatrists
with a sales pitch approach based on eye glass
prescription in 1979. They packaged their
prescription orthotic in bright colours, adapted it for
various markets, ensured the paperwork looked
professional and delivered a product efficiently.
Although both directors were from a podiatry
background, Langer opened its market to other
groups and trained anyone they felt they could
validate and promote their product. The success of
their marketing strategy changed the face of orthotic
manufacture and presentation in the UK forever. As
a marketing exercise this example is important
because it shows that Langer understood its market.
It targeted it with a message that could be
understood and appealed to many who did not want
to spend hours pressing plastic, grinding and
polishing, and breathing in methyl methacrylate
fumes. Over the years many companies started to

support podiatrists in other areas using similar marketing tools to Langer.

Patient chairs - Both the NHS and private sector originally used heavy cumbersome throne like chairs used by patients. The design was adorned with heavy ribbed tred steps, tubular metal arm rests and a non-reclinable back. The image of podiatry looked better when the patient reclined in a moulded space age dental type couch, but these soon became expensive. A new design called Akron was made available but without the contoured finish. Based around the physiotherapy couch this offered a smart alternative to the old fashioned plinth couch. As with Pampers the cost influenced where coin would be spent. When it was realised that it was vital to recline seats to allow for CPR, the old fashioned chairs became obsolete. Opportunity dominated and justified the reason for using a product with a multi-purpose function.

Padding- The mainstay treatment for foot pain, callus, ulcers, hammer toes and bunions was a combination of dressings using felt, foam and fleece. The material varied in thickness, colour and density. Podiatrists originally trained for hours cutting out shapes. When Silipos products arrived all the the key stone podiatric skills reduced.

The last example covers a condition most of us have treated at some time in our career. Love them or hate them, warts are a feature of podiatry. The recipe of corns, warts, bunions and hammer toes are beloved by comedians or journalists. In his 1845 publication, surgeon chiropodist Lewis Durlacher a wordy title to his book, although his wart treatment appears under general management:

> A treatise on corns, bunions, the diseases of the nails and the general management of the foot.

Management of warts - The idea that acids are appropriate for managing viral skin infections (warts) is unreliable. What works for one patient does not work for another. Risks from caustic toxicity and alarming reactions were common. Controllable microwave methods were introduced to treat warts influencing the market slowly but surely. The product can be packaged in terms of efficiency, clean delivery, lower side effects, which are all potentially better for the patient.

Podiatrist Ivan Bristow has developed his brand through skin pathology in feet. The difference between Bristow and others is that he markets to podiatrists rather than patients.

Sale's technique

One method described by a well known US podiatrist was to show no emotion when selling orthoses. He tested the market on the spot and adjusted his sales pitch.

> "If I thought the patient was good for it I would look him in the eye and say the orthotic was

179

$150.00 bucks. If he showed no reaction I would
then say, *for each foot*!"

This is opportunistic and unfair but such approaches
to business are well known. *Make it up as you go!* It
is important to have a tariff that you can refer to and
this should be available in cases of dispute. As
Osgo's Tony Gavin mentioned, all your processes
should be documented.

Conferences, Meetings and Journals

How do we find out what's going on? If you are at
the cutting edge of research, then of course this
provides an opportunity to reflect academically on
the market. Almost every research paper is seeking
a new angle to prove, disprove and make a change
to clinical practice. Few podiatrists are engaged in
this activity so this leaves the larger percentage of
podiatry sifting information.

Conferences and meetings are important as this is
where we talk. Communication and sharing is vital
for us all to move forward. A professional journal is
important, but podiatrists, like many now prefer
social media or electronic systems over paper.

In much the same way this book has also adopted an
e-book format. When Linda Merriman and I were
first commissioned to write *Clinical Skills and
Assessment of the Lower Limb*, the idea that a book
could be delivered electronically was something we

did not think could happen back in 1994. Look how much that market has changed.

A final chapter covering advertising tips has been included as website development is important. The medium is both popular and accessible.

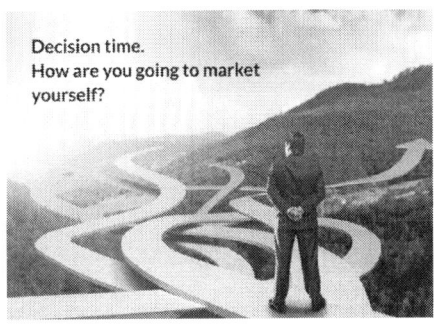

Decision time.
How are you going to market yourself?

11. Website advertising & Useful Tips

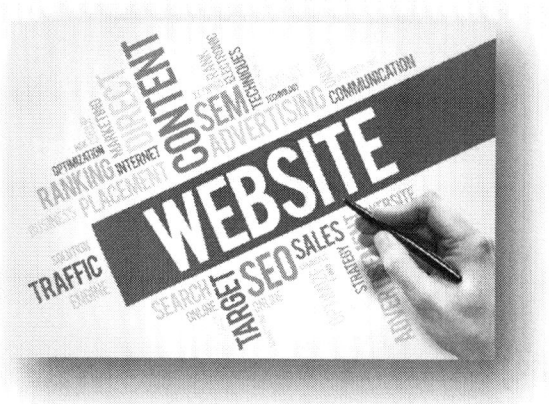

Shutterstock/dizain

LET'S LOOK AT THE POTENTIAL

It is not possible to recommend any particular site as it must suite your budget and need. I have set out some criteria that you might find helpful but if you want to promote your business seriously then consider a website. Having stated the advertising potential of a website, this medium also plays an important delivery in foot health promotion. In reality you will need a website at least for information dissemination which will lead to the conclusion within this chapter. Websites can be linked to Facebook, LinkedIn, Twitter and Instagram as examples of common social media platforms. Paid advertising can be purchased to drive people to your website using Facebook and LinkedIn. In this age of modern fast communication, you cannot avoid creating a web base to support your practice. You should be able to edit your website. and buddied up to a mail delivery system will offer a valuable mechanism for staying in touch with clients.

I use Mail Chimp presently but there are many such products with free start up packages. You can serve a population of at least 1000 subscribers for free. This helps you keeping in touch, create a newsletter and so forth.

When you first consider all of these products it appears as if you are in a little boat in a rough sea not knowing which wave to steer through first. Start simple and build. Rome (as they say) was not built in a day and you will get things wrong at the start. Who doesn't! What matters is that you learn from your mistakes and improve. I learn something almost every day and find keeping up with change is demanding. It is necessary to navigate to around the tricksters where websites are vulnerable. Spam bots and automated intruders try to help you improve your website, and there are others who send inappropriate material.

(1) No Website Yet. Have you considered the benefits?

- Advertising in your community allows new clients to search for your style of practice.
- Providing a method for efficient booking.
- Promoting your service allows you to reach the right clientele to work with your preferred expertise.
- Attaching information can save excessive costs in producing paperwork.
- Provides a cost effective way of keeping your information updated, colourful and geared to your own image. Note that you need to put in some effort
- Websites need time to maintain currency.
- Task in administrative time daily – weekly depending upon the type of website that you run.
- Edit and upgrade information material to show that it is current.
- Update hyperlinking and check it works from time to time.

COSTS & SERVICES

You will need to pay for the website, organise and register your name as a **domain.** This has to be licensed annually with a fee. The costs are offset with reduced advertising elsewhere. If you pay someone this can be included in a monthly fee. Maintaining your site, dealing with back up and ensuring it does not fail are vital. People will hack into your site. My own site has filters to remove abusive hits. At other times you will find people writing to you suggesting that they can improve your search engine optimization (SEO). Be careful and don't get drawn in and delete these e-mails. Stick with the company or person you have elected to organise the administration of your website.

Clearly costs can vary but the best advice is to look around, find someone local and definitely in the UK if you are British, likewise in the USA, stick to US providers. Recommendations are helpful but check out the web designer's testimonials. Ask for fees and what they entail before making a decision. Professional sites will publish costs. You will want someone friendly and at the end of a phone or e-mail. In 2020 prices you are going to need to spend above £10 a month with a potential of around £25 a month for a useful package. Of course the costs can escalate in terms of what you might wish to achieve. The annual plan therefore may typically come in at £500 – £1000. This might sound a big outlay but if you are serious about your business then it is an essential method for today's climate in which to promote a viable service.

(2) You already have a website?

Check list
- Does it serve to advertise your address, clinic location, times of opening and bookings?
- Does it say what you do?
- Does it have one or more pages?
- Are you selling anything on your website? If not do you want to?

A static page may work well for your business but interactive pages do so much more. Analytics provide a breakdown of activity. Sites such as WordPress build this into their basic packages. Other actions to consider for your website:

- Set up more pages.
- Make a page up dedicated to products.
- Set up a features page of the key topics of health you cover and treatment methods.
- Not reaching clients? Review search engine optimization.

(3) You have no direct website ownership?

- If you don't have a website how do you advertise?
- Does someone else promote your brand?
- Are you supported by a bigger brand website from the independent sector to NHS?
- Does this work for you?

If you work in the NHS, you may wish to negotiate your departmental brand. So often this is not that well developed and a golden opportunity for promotion is lost.

My independent hospitals had websites and advertised me as a specialist but the data and profile was basic and did not allow me to expand beyond this elementary information, let alone enable me to edit my material directly. Changing anything meant an e-mail, delay and then an adjustment days or weeks later. This is not good for a busy practice. Now if you had your own website you can use the link or uniform resource locator address (URL) and have it attached to the hospital site which expands your reach and allows you to develop in the direction you want to go. More clients, more profile and easier ways to disseminate information.

Actions: Assuming that you want to use a website, make sure that you can control content.

(4) Want to do more?

- Find a do-it-yourself website builder OR find a web builder who can help you if this first idea is outside of your comfort zone.
- Start simple. Create a landing page with a basic advert.
- Single pages are cost effective and easy to maintain. Trial your site for 1-3 months but make sure you can add pages later if possible even if only to promote information.

 There are plenty of website products available. Sonder (UK) used here only as an example will offer you different types of support. Just search for yourself and compare prices and packages. Attaching documents, images and video clips may also be important for your site but be cautious as some sites may not handle all features. Start with basic packages but if you want broader services you will have to invest more.

(5) Key features after your landing page

There are areas you will need to consider beyond a simple static landing page. Remember web sites are selected with a mouse click. Advertise your web

address 'everywhere' and seek out links to your
website on other sites. Put it on headed paper, e-
mails, business cards.
 Other actions you might consider
- Images
- Pages for testimonials
- Information on products (if you are selling items)
- Health information on the foot (see sections 6-7)

 Images are powerful communicators and quality
images ideally should be licensed which means
outlay. There are free sites but because this is a
commercial proposition, do be careful not to use an
imprinted 'stock' picture without license. Take you
own photos and make sure you have a professional
head shot of yourself. Testimonials are powerful
and I have considered this subject in *chapter 9:
Logos, Brand, Strap line.*

Information about products or selling products from
your website is something you can consider for
additional income. The probity of selling in
healthcare is not a subject for this book but should
be considered as part of your professional ethics. A
well tested product that serves a purpose is fair
game but the idea of making an unfair killing may
not be akin the spirit of good practice.

(6) Selling a foot health commodity
Patients will search locally to make a decision who
to go to, although many will use personal
recommendations. Use of Yellow Pages or a
professional register might find you. Your website

should have a quality professional head shot of you in good light and a clean landing page.

Ideally design a strap line to sell yourself. This should be short at around 5 words. Ensure part of the landing page tells the enquirer what you do. Keep this simple as well as use easy to understand language. Remember that the landing page should encourage people to read more. 'Clickable' areas can be used such as buttons designed to guide someone to a heading that provides more information. e.g ABOUT YOU. What do you offer treatment wise? A bit about podiatry and the profession can be helpful. Make sure that you use headings to split up the areas of your work. Design all of your good intentions on paper first using one page per message to create on the website.

LINK INFORMATION TO YOUR SITE

Content writing
It is unlikely that you will find anyone keyed into podiatry writing on your behalf except those who desire to write about the subject of feet. Try to look around and find someone who might allow you to share material first. If not, try writing your own material which gives you better control of what you might want. If you want to develop your own information site but have little time, then use a link for specific conditions to ensure established quality for your site. ConsultingFootPain material is free to link to but it should not be copied without citation

and acknowledgement or altered without permission. Write at the bottom of the page or where you intend to place the information;

Information accessed on 21/5/2020 Original article written by DRT or whoever using full title and name.

Content marketing and SEO development can be purchased professionally and is easily found using search engines. One site mentioned earlier was Reedsy. It might be worth saying a little bit about Reedsy as I have several years experience with them. The landing page will tell you that they produce beautiful books but what you are looking for is a writer. The marketing sections of most use will be publicity, marketing and website. Access is all free and you can put in your requirements, select from the professionals listed and invite usually 5 to bid for your work. You accept or decline as needed and agree a fee. The fees are taken in instalments depending upon how much you spend. This should all be geared to non-fiction work. Reedsy ensure all work is professionally conducted and like PayPal act as arbiters and offers some financial protection.

Elsewhere, content writing typically is advertised as starting from around £30/page. There is a whole market out there waiting to help if you need it. I will certainly be happy to assist any podiatrist but would work as any freelance would. Do use links to reliable information sites. I talked about this in earlier chapters and make the comment that patient information is not always appropriate from the professional organisations. By using reliable sites that you should be able to vet for yourself will save you having to write more than a brief introduction. Majority of information that you can access needs no copyright permission if it is linked up. Use the link and copy this into your own page. Pick sites written by podiatrists, orthopaedic surgeons, physiotherapists and health journalists. Those with professional qualifications and past publication credits are my top group and I ignore content where the information ends in a hard sell.

(7) Setting up information

If you are used to writing, fine you can do all of this yourself. Remember that your web designer cannot help write professional material. Draft it out first and then import the text and build around the design.

Leaflets created for different treatment programmes are useful and support the idea of consent (Tollafield 2019). While I have designed numerous (A4) sheets, I took the key conditions such as IGTN, steroid injections, surgery (generic), corns and bunions and made the information into open up trifold leaflets. These were glossy and colourful to give my patients. However, as time progressed I decided where patients were able to use my website this offered a better platform for my clinical information. Patients could then be redirected to my website and my clinical notes also recorded this advice. Designing articles became a valuable asset and I soon wrote articles about patients and found patients willing to post testimonials. I still engage in this practice and some can be found on my webpages now as open access articles for the public.

Websites are fun but for most busy practitioners it is part of the business that is rarely exploited fully. So what can you do? Support your website and practice with leaflets.

PRODUCE YOUR OWN LEAFLET

If you cannot find a leaflet from source, then design one using many of the on-line publishing sites. Some are based abroad but again try to find local printers who can deliver glossy leaflets in A5 or the popular DL (dimension leaflet). By using local sources, you can discuss how best to produce copy e.g. should you allow images to bleed or have margins. Bleed is a term that relates to the pictures or illustrations and text not having a margin and so will run to the edge of the page. Pictures can offer a better appearance when they consume the whole page. In contrast, the titled e-book version of this book included the use of bleed for each chapter page but in the paperback version bleed is not used. You can design the cover, import images, and making the appearance personal. The costs can be contained and you can order from 25-50 upwards as well as download a sample copy for proof reading.

Designs and laying out your leaflet (formatting) requires modest skills well within the range of most people. It is always a question of the time that is available to undertake such tasks. Leaflets can also act as glossy business cards. These can be stored in

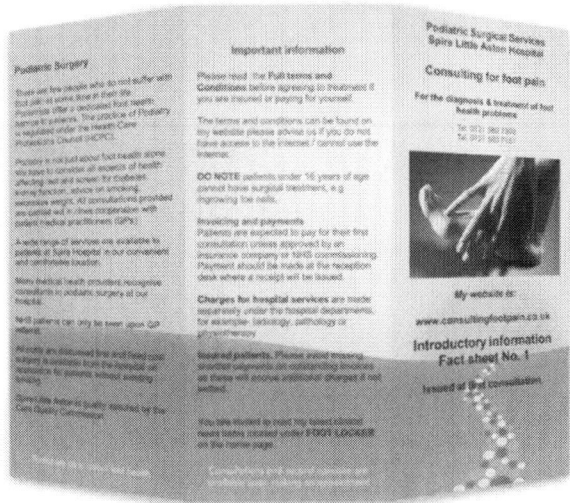

accessible racks so patients can browse whilst in the waiting room or pass onto friends and family.

Example of a trifold leaflet. The front picture was not set up to bleed to the edges

The leaflet above was my main practice leaflet setting out conditions and other information. I started using this system as far back as 2009. It came as a trifold and allowed me to print a sample off to check for spelling and grammar before purchasing in batches. This meant I only needed to order small numbers so I could update the leaflet before each order. Print on demand has become the best method to obtain printed material. The logos and pictures used could be imported and the style and colour selected. The two tone background came from the printer's stock which matched my needs at the time.

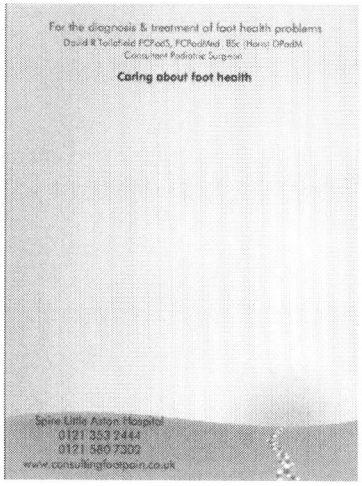

Do note the information on the tear off pad is no longer valid. You can add pens, and design professional pads that patients can take away all in the same colour scheme. Most on-line printing firms today offer other products from mugs to clothing that can carry logos and businesses. Of course there is a balance between what is appropriate and what will work from a professional view point.

Articles written on websites make great resources for your practice. The link begins with the http:// and then the specific code unique for the article.

Podiatrists can assist patients with peripheral neuropathy in two ways. Recognising the extent of numbness by testing sensations with special fibres and providing advice how to care for the foot. Patients who have other risk factors such as diabetes mellitus and obesity, as well as those with vitamin B_{12} anaemia are at a higher risk of developing peripheral neuropathy. For example, some cancer drugs affect blood sugar levels of diabetic patients which can affect the nerves further.

Burning

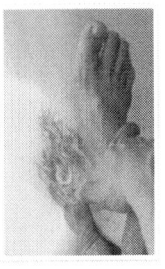

It is relatively common for patients to complain of a burning sensation in their hands and feet and some have found this to be so severe that they have had to take morphine lollipops to help manage the pain. Symptoms may include a sensation as if wearing a glove or stocking that can extend to the knee. The severity depends on the dosage, frequency and length of each treatment cycle. peripheral neuropathy negatively affects awareness of what position each joint is in. This is called proprioception and the messages to the brain are interrupted affecting how patients move. Mobility associated with walking is affected as the patient can't walk comfortably and abnormal pressure is created. This increases the risk of neuropathic ulceration and infection developing. Your podiatrist will be able to monitor the risk, provide support or padding to reduce the ulcer forming and advice on how to handle the burning sensation.

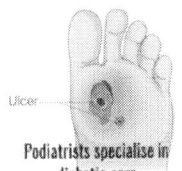

Podiatrists specialise in diabetic care

Numbness affect walking patterns

The style of walking changes so that increased pressure results in certain areas on the foot, causing footwear to feel uncomfortable or painful. This might sound strange when numbness is present but not all sensations disappear, creating confusion for the patient. Elderly patients particularly experience such symptoms

Solutions and help for cancer patients

Example, http://consultingfootpain.co.uk/how-can-podiatrists-help-with-peripheral-neuropathy/

(8) Do You Need Help?
While I don't provide any support for websites I like to encourage podiatrists to link clinical

information and articles which can be designed as part of their own website. For single platform page sites, you can link your site to CFP with a dedicated article to your practice. This can be shared openly with the public at no cost. Such publicity benefits all parties. We can take raw information and turn it into a useful article. Many podiatrists write on social media platforms where their information can be helpful to others. This information can be harnessed into a professional newsletter, article, blog as well as leaflet. So, if you need help write to me and maybe I can help or maybe not.

And finally ....

To ignore social media and the potential brought by a website is like ignoring on-line banking or sticking to cheques when the world around you uses electronic transactions. Few can fight change but we cannot remain successful without exploiting our brand efficiently and effectively. Ask yourselves this,

DO I WANT TO EXPAND, CHANGE FROM BRAND CHIROPODY OR AM I COMFORTABLE BECAUSE MY DIARY IS FULLY BOOKED FOR WEEKS?

Thank you for reading my book, if you feel you can leave feedback I would be grateful.

My correspondence address is davidt@busypencilcase.com

12. References

REFERENCES BEHIND SELLING FOOT HEALTH AS PODIATRY

How do we package Podiatry? Was launched in a leaflet (November 2019) at the Annual College of Podiatry conference[22] and available to signed-up Newsfeed readers.
Tollafield DR. We should always have an opportunity to change attitudes. 2019 (8):46-50
Tollafield DR. *How do we package Podiatry?* Burden of Foot Health. Part 1. 2019 2(12):72-75
Tollafield DR. *How do we package Podiatry?* How can we learn from looking at the whole canvas? Part 2. 2019 2(12):77-80
Tollafield DR. *How do we package Podiatry?* Giving credit to our brand Part 3. 2020 3(1):1-5
Tollafield DR. *How do we package Podiatry?* Logo, brand, strap line. Part 4. 2020 3(2):6-10
Tollafield DR. *How do we package Podiatry?* How do we deliver the message? Part 5. 2020.3(2):11-15

LINKS TO PROFESSIONAL BODIES & OTHER INFORMATION ON FOOT HEALTH
British Orthopaedic Foot & Ankle Society deals with patient information and provides views on other organisations
https://www.bofas.org.uk/Patient-Information
College of Podiatry common foot conditions are covered
https://cop.org.uk/foot-health/common-foot-problems/

---

[22] Written under ***Reflective Podiatric Practice***, published by Busypencilcase Communications Ltd.

Institute of Chiropody & Podiatry promotes footcare advice
https://iocp.org.uk/footcare-advice/
Osgo Promoting podiatry https://www.osgo.co.uk/product-category/promoting-podiatry/

CHAPTER 1
WHAT'S IN A NAME?

Gavin, Tony Independent Podiatry. A Personal Journey.
Landscape Interviews. April 14 2020
Durlacher, L A Concise Treatise on Corns, bunions and the disorder of nails with advice for the general management of the feet. London: Simpkin, Marshall & Co.1858

CHAPTER 2
COMMUNICATION WITH PATIENTS

Beckman HB, Frankel RM. The effect of physician behaviour on the collection of data. Ann.Intern. Med. 1984;101(5):692-6
Burt, J, Abel, G, Elmore, N, Campbell, J, Roland, M, Benson, J, Silverman, J. Assessing communication quality of consultations in primary care: initial reliability of the Global Consultation Rating Scale, based on the Calgary-Cambridge Guide to the Medical Interview. Doi:10.11.1136/bmjopen-2013-004339
College of Podiatry. www.PASCOM-10 –Resources. Open access
Hood IS, Kilmartin TE, Tollafield DR. The effect of Podiatric day case surgery on the need for NHS chiropody treatment. The Foot 1994; 4:155-158
Kindelan, K, Kent G. Concordance between patients' information preferences and general practitioners' perceptions/ Psychol Health. 1987;1(4):399-409
McKinley, RK, Middleton, JF. What do patients want from doctors? Content analysis of written patient agendas for consultation. Br. J. Gen Pract. 1999;49(447):796-800
Siddique, H GP Appointments Should Be Five Minutes Longer Says BMA.
https://www.theguardian.com/society/2016/aug/28/doctor-appointments-15-minutes-bma-overweight-population

Silverman, J, Kurtz, S, Draper, J. Skills for communicating with patients (third ed.) CRC Press Taylor & Francis Group 2013

CHAPTER 3
HOW TO COMMUNICATE

Beckman HB, Frankel RM. The effect of physician behaviour on the collection of data. Ann.Intern. Med. 1984;101(5):692-6
Campitelli, N Surgery for Morton's Neuroma.
https://www.youtube.com/watch?v=GrFS-67_ZCc 21 Nov. 2013
Cowley E, Lepesis, V The SOAPIER Model in podiatric musculo assessment and management. Podiatry Now. Sept. 2018;8-10
Kilmartin TE, Tollafield DR, Jones L. Clinical clerking for Podiatrists. Br. J. Podiatric Medicine and Surgery 1991; 3:2-5
Seymour CA, Introduction to Clinical Clerking. Cambridge University Press 1984
Silverman, J, Kurtz, S, Draper, J. Skills for communicating with patients (third ed.) CRC Press Taylor & Francis Group 2013
White, J, Levinson, W, Roter, D. 'Oh by the way': the closing moments of the medical interview. J. Gen Int Med. 1994; 9:24-8
Tollafield D R Making those decisions about our profession as a career. Podiatry Now. 2019; July:16-17
Office for National Statistics
(https://www.ons.gov.uk/businessindustryandtrade/itandintern etindustry/bulletins/internetusers/2016)

CHAPTER 4
INFORMATION CONVERSION

Barnes, A, Littlewood, K, Harle, J, Beecroft, C, Burnside, J, Wheeler, T, Selwyn
Farndon L, Vernon DW, Parry A. What is the evidence for the continuation of core podiatry services in the NHS: A review of foot surveys? Br J Podiatry. 2006; 9:89–94.Farndon, L, Godfrey, E (Ed.) Raise Your Rating. Podiatry Now. 2020; May:20-25

Harrison-Blount, M, Nester, C, Williams, A. The changing Landscape of professional practice in podiatry, lessons to be learned from other professions about barriers to change – a narrative view. JFAR. 2019:12-23

Laxton, C Clinical Audit of Forefoot Surgery performed by Registered Medical Practitioners and Podiatrists. J. Public Health Medicine 1995.17:311-317

Morris, S, Walters, SJ. Clinical audit of core podiatry treatment in the NHS. JFAR.2009;2:7 doi:10.1186/1757-1146-2-7

Noakes, K 2015 https://www.how2become.com/blog/good-paying-jobs-that-nobody-wants/

Office of National Statistics. Internet Users in the UK 2019 https://www.ons.gov.uk/businessindustryandtrade/itandinternetindustry/bulletins/internetusers/2019

Tarr, I Landscape Interview Diabetes and podiatry. April 2020

CHAPTER 5
OPTIMISING INFORMATION THROUGH IMAGE

Tollafield DR May 2020
http://consultingfootpain.co.uk/what-can-i-do-to-help-myself/
This covers bunion pad (6.15), Mobilising the first toe (3.04) and The Fan Strap (5.20)

CHAPTER 6
THE BURDEN OF FOOT HEALTH

Bowen, C. Future Academic and miscellaneous Podiatry. Landscape Interview. April 29 2020

Bowen, C Addressing the Burden of Rheumatic and Musculoskeletal Foot & Ankle Pain. 2019 May 2019 YouTube https://www.youtube.com/watch?v=kQ0OSmbQFmE&t=109s

Bowen C. Encounters for foot and ankle pain in UK primary care: a population-based cohort study of CPRD data. Br J Gen Pract. 2019 Jun;69(683):e422-e429. doi: 10.3399/bjgp19X703817. Epub 2019 May 20. PubMed PMID: 31109927; PubMed Central PMCID: PMC6532799.

Dando C, Bacon D, Borthwick A, Redmond A, Bowen CJ. Stakeholder views of podiatry services in the UK for people living with arthritis: a qualitative investigation. *In preparation April 2020.*

Edwards K, Borthwick A, McCulloch L, Redmond AC, Ferguson R, Culliford D, Prieto-Alhambra D, Pinedo-Villanueva R, Delmestri A, Arden N, Pinedo-Villanueva R, Arden NK, Bowen CJ. Evidence for current recommendations concerning the management of foot health for people with chronic long-term conditions: a systematic review. *Journal of Foot and Ankle Research.* (2017) 10:51. (22 Nov).

McCulloch L, Borthwick A, Redmond A, Edwards K, O'Neill, G, Ross, M, Burden of care: An important concept for nurses. Healthcare for Women International. 2011; 12:111-121 https://doi.org/10.1080/07399339109515931

Pinedo-Villanueva R, Prieto-Alhambra D, Judge A, Arden NK, Bowen CJ. UK podiatrists' experiences of podiatry services for people living with arthritis: a qualitative investigation. J Foot Ankle Res. 2018 Jun 5; 11:27. doi: 10.1186/s13047-018-0262-5. eCollection 2018. PubMed PMID: 29928316; PubMed Central PMCID: PMC5989380.

Farndon, L, Concannon, M, Stephenson, J A survey to investigate the association of pain, foot disability and quality of life with corns. Journal of Foot and Ankle Research (2015) 8:70 doi 10.1186/s13047-015-0131-4

Tarr, I Diabetes and Podiatry. Landscape Interview. April 2020

Tollafield DR Myths & Facts. Ingrowing toenail. 2019; Aug 10 http://consultingfootpain.co.uk/myths-facts-ingrowing-toenail/

Williams, A. Footwear Assessment and Management. Podiatry Now. Continuous Professional Development Supplement. 2006; May: S1-S8

CHAPTER 7
LOOKING AT THE WHOLE CANVAS

Afni Shah-Hamilton The Role of Podiatrists in Cancer Care. Part 1. Early identification & Diagnosis. Busypencilcase Communications Ltd. 2020;3(2):16-20

Sonia C Gregory. Building a brand that aligns with your purpose. Freshsparks. Accessed 10 April 2020 https://freshsparks.com/successful-brand-building-process/
Tollafield, DR, Merriman, LM, Clinical Skills in Treating the foot. Tollafield, DR, Surgery and the Foot Churchill-Livingstone. 1997:108
Tollafield, DR, Clinical Skills in Treating the Foot. Turner, WA, Merriman, LM, Surgery and the Foot Churchill-Livingstone. 2005:122

CHAPTER 8
HOW DO WE DELIVER THE MESSAGE?

NHS Link to an example of a health condition: chilblains https://www.nhs.uk/conditions/chilblains/
NICE Link to history https://www.nice.org.uk/about/who-we-are/history-of-nice
www.FootEducation.com A North American foot and ankle patient database
Tollafield DR. What should you ask from a factsheet? Footlocker: April 2019 (http://consultingfootpain.co.uk/what-should-you-ask-from-a-factsheet/)
Taylor, NG, Tollafield DR, Rees S. Does patient satisfaction with foot surgery change over time? The Foot 2008;18(2):68-74

CHAPTER 9
LOGO, BRAND, STRAP LINE

Bergman, Eric. 5 Steps to conquer 'Death by Powerpoint'. Changing the world one conversation at a time. Petticoat Creek Press Inc. 2012 Step #3. Minimizing visual aids. Pp85 - 87
Catherine Kaputa (2012) You are a Brand. Brealey Publishing. Second ed.
Hope, C, Dixon, H The Rallying Cry that may have worked too well. The Daily Telegraph. 20 May 2020:14
Raise Your Rating. *House of Commons Podiatry: staff: written question – 18581 April 2020* in Podiatry Now 2020; May:21

Sonia C Gregory. Building a brand that aligns with your purpose. Freshsparks. Accessed 10 April 2020
https://freshsparks.com/successful-brand-building-process/

CHAPTER 10
GIVING CREDIT TO OUR BRAND

Kings Fund. Helen Stokes-Lampard: Social prescribing and the current NHS landscape May 18, 2017.
https://www.kingsfund.org.uk/audio-video/helen-stokes-lampard-social-prescribing

CHAPTER 11
WEBSITE ADVERTISING & USEFUL TIPS

10 top tip Self Build Designs
https://www.top10bestwebsitebuilders.co.uk/
Tollafield DR Podiatry and the Changing Face of Consent Podiatry. Podiatry Review. Issue (CPD pull out) Autumn 2019 pp17-20.

THE LANDSCAPE INTERVIEWS

These interviews relate to the project title of another book (in preparation) covering podiatry as a career. Interviews were extensively used by the author and included in this book.

Index

Foot Health Journey Books
from the same author

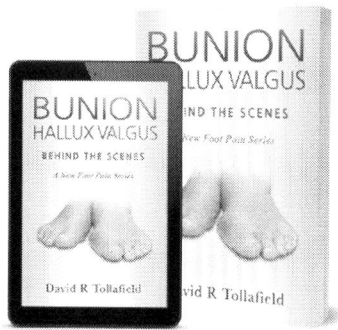

Bunion. Hallux Valgus.
Behind the Scenes

… I had to scratch around the internet looking at blogs, which mainly were American. In fact, had I read your book I may well have saved myself some money. Your book is extremely well written and I would highly recommend anyone considering surgery to read this first. There was more post-op information than anything that I could find! - *N. Harvey, Patient*

…I really wish a comprehensive book like this had been available prior to my first surgery…This 'warts and all' approach provides some very honest, frank and practical information and certainly would have prepared me for what lay ahead. - *J. Homer, Patient*

Foot Health Journey Books

from the same author

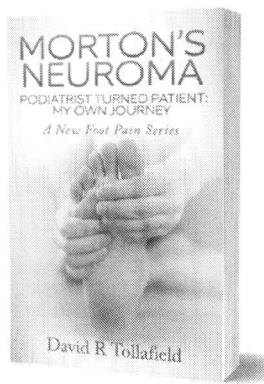

Morton's Neuroma.
Podiatrist Turned Patient: My own Journey

...Very easy to understand ... I would have found it helpful to have something like this as I was on google and wanted as much information as possible prior to surgery. -
Mrs Jenny Norton, Patient

...this book is very accessible and easily understandable by the lay reader/patient (due to its clear, simple and concise language) without losing any of its medical scientific value... - **Dr Marius Vintella**

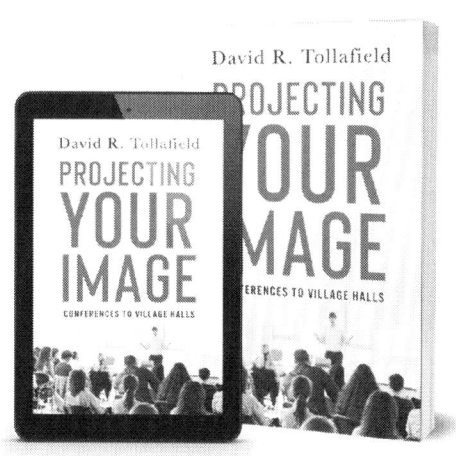

Projecting Your Image

Laced with humour that reinforces the message and illustrated throughout with highly relevant case studies, David Tollafield's book will guide you every step of the way to transform your dull and mundane lectures into transactional events that will keep your audiences alert, awake and, most of all, motivated. - **Roy Jones, Professional Educator retired, South West England.**

Also see the companion to this book and manual *Thinking as We Build* offering tips on building your PowerPoint talk currently only available in paperback.

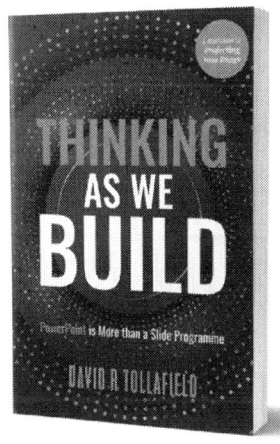

Thinking as We Build

Thinking as We Build - PowerPoint is more than a slide Programme. The perfect companion to *Projecting Your Image*, providing the nuts and bolts when building your talk. The illustrated text amalgamates a manual of how to use PowerPoint with the process of designing a talk that you can be proud of. Easy to use and follow with diagrams and screen shots alongside structured examples of how to achieve the best from your slide deck

'Reflecting on his own mistakes allows the reader to relate more accurately to the key points made in this book. The book was well organised making it easier to dip in and out as needed. The quotes used from many seasoned sources were both relevant and emphasised the point being made in each chapter,' **Professor David Pratt, (former) Director Bioengineering, Birmingham**

Printed in Great Britain
by Amazon